Sandra Dubs

MY WHOLEFOOD COMMUNITY PLANT BASED COOK BOOK

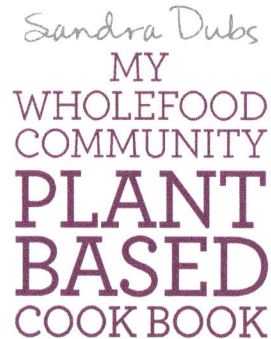

Sandra Dubs
MY WHOLEFOOD COMMUNITY PLANT BASED COOK BOOK

This edition printed in 2022
Self-published in Australia by Sandra Dubs
www.mywholefoodcommunity.com

All rights are reserved. No part of this publication may be reproduced, stored in a retrieval system or transmitted in any form of by any means, electronic, mechanical, photocopying, recording or otherwise without prior permission from the author.

The information contained in these pages is not intended nor implied to be a substitute for professional medical advice. It is provided for educational purposes only.
The author may not be held responsible for any action or claim resulting from the use of information within this book. The moral right of the author has been asserted.

Copyright © Sandra Dubs My Wholefood Community™ 2019.

ISBN 978-0-648-11350-8 Australia

Written and compiled by Sandra Dubs.
Design by The Hive Design.
Editing by Stephanie Heriot AE.
Photography by Emmanuel Santos.

Catalogue-in-Publications data is available from the National Library of Australia.

Dedicated to the ones I love

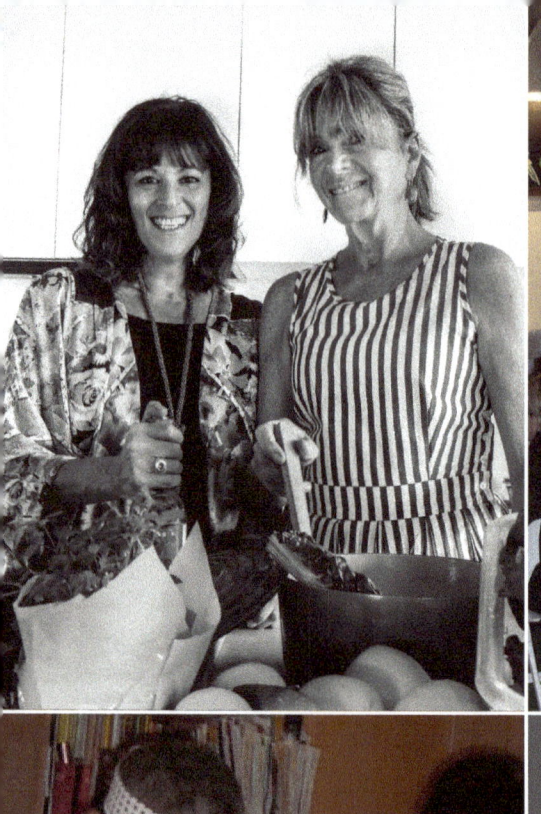
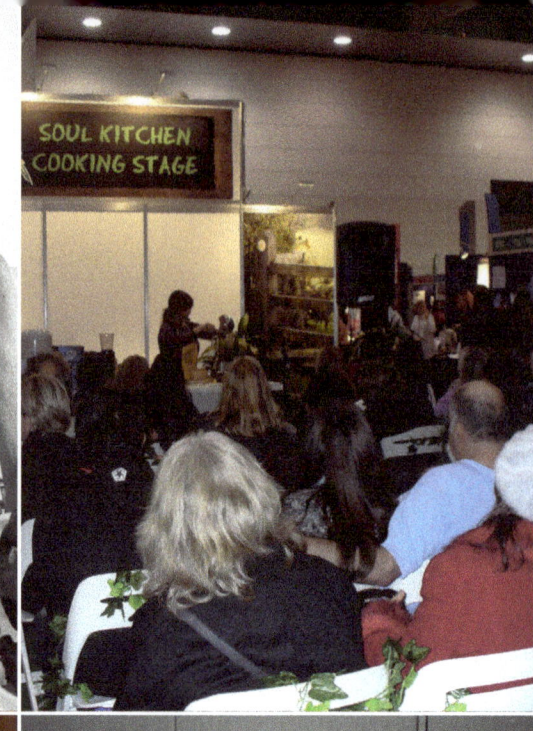
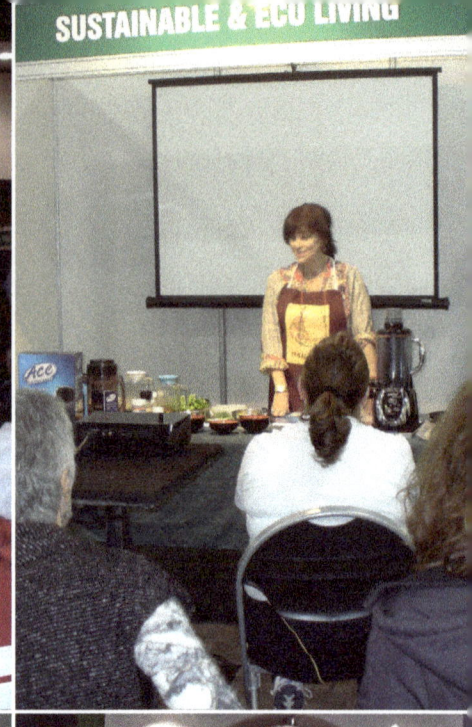
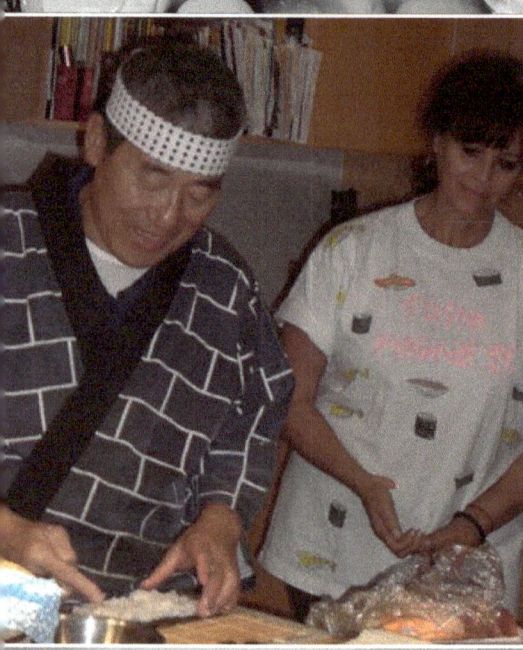
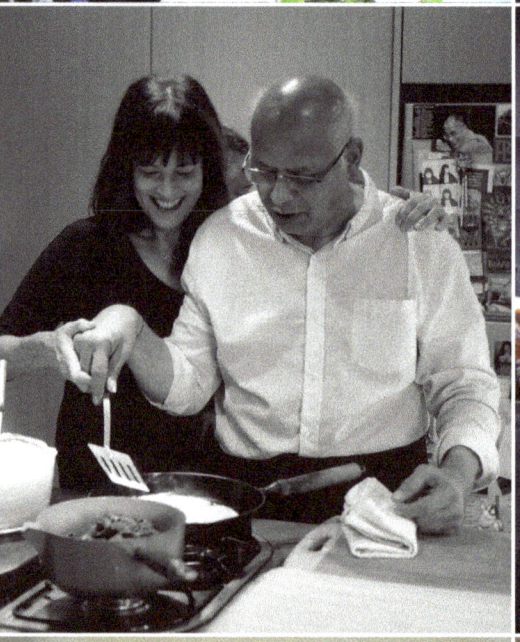
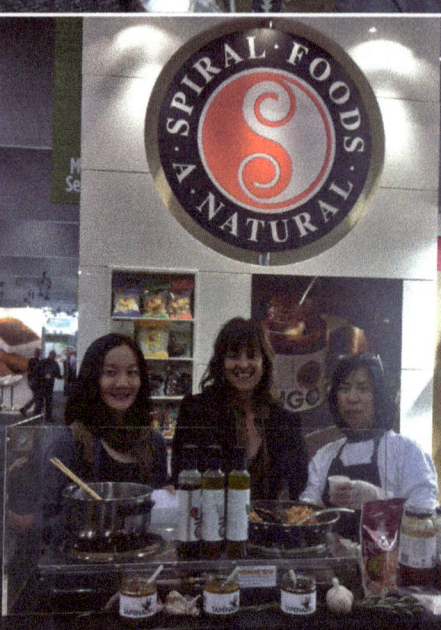
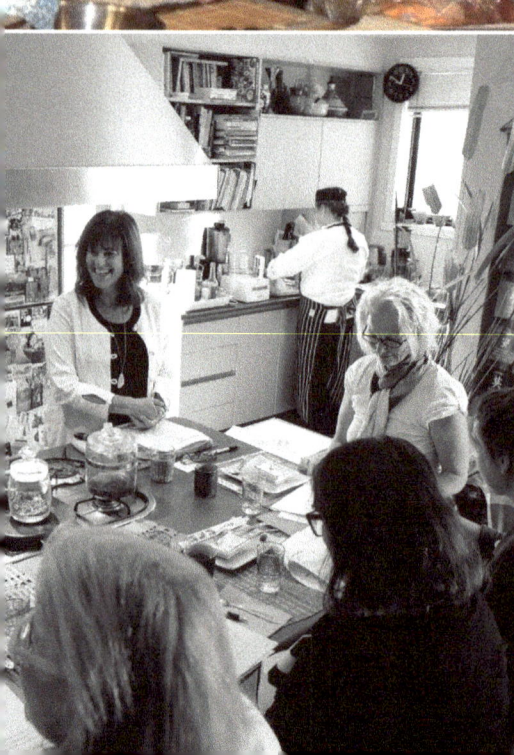
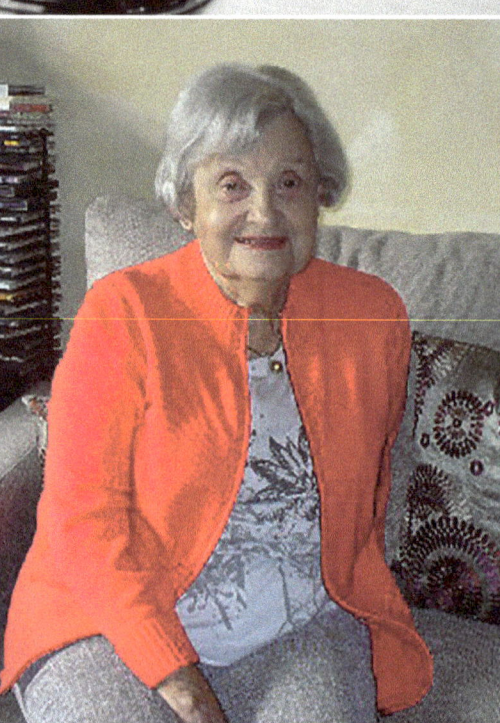
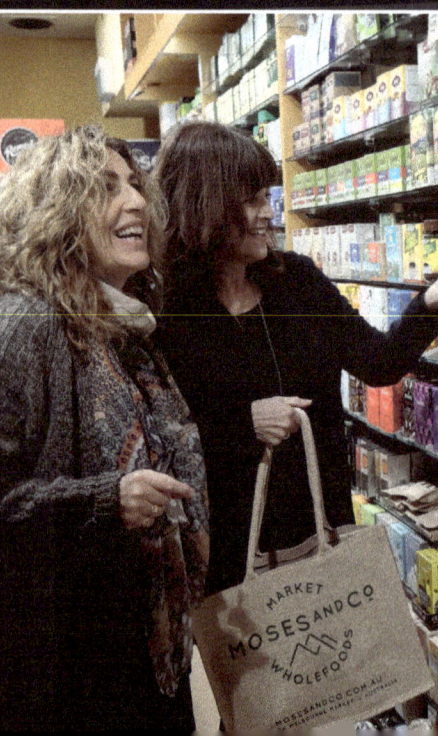

I am part of a wonderful wholefood community, and now you are too!

My Wholefood Community

This book reflects the wonderful feedback and support that I have received from people who have participated in my classes over the years and from clients who have come for nutritional support.

I am happy and rewarded in so many ways to have been involved in the plant-based wholefood movement for the past 35 years. I continue to learn and share by running cooking classes and presenting workshops and seminars on food as medicine and nutrition for wellbeing, as well as consulting and creating health-supportive wellbeing programs for corporate and private clients. Enjoying health-supportive wholefoods and using foods as medicines is a support to many and naturally to me.

I acknowledge and thank the many suppliers of organic and natural foods whom I have known for so long and who continue to support my work and lifestyle. I am proud to include them in this book.

This is my great purpose in life.

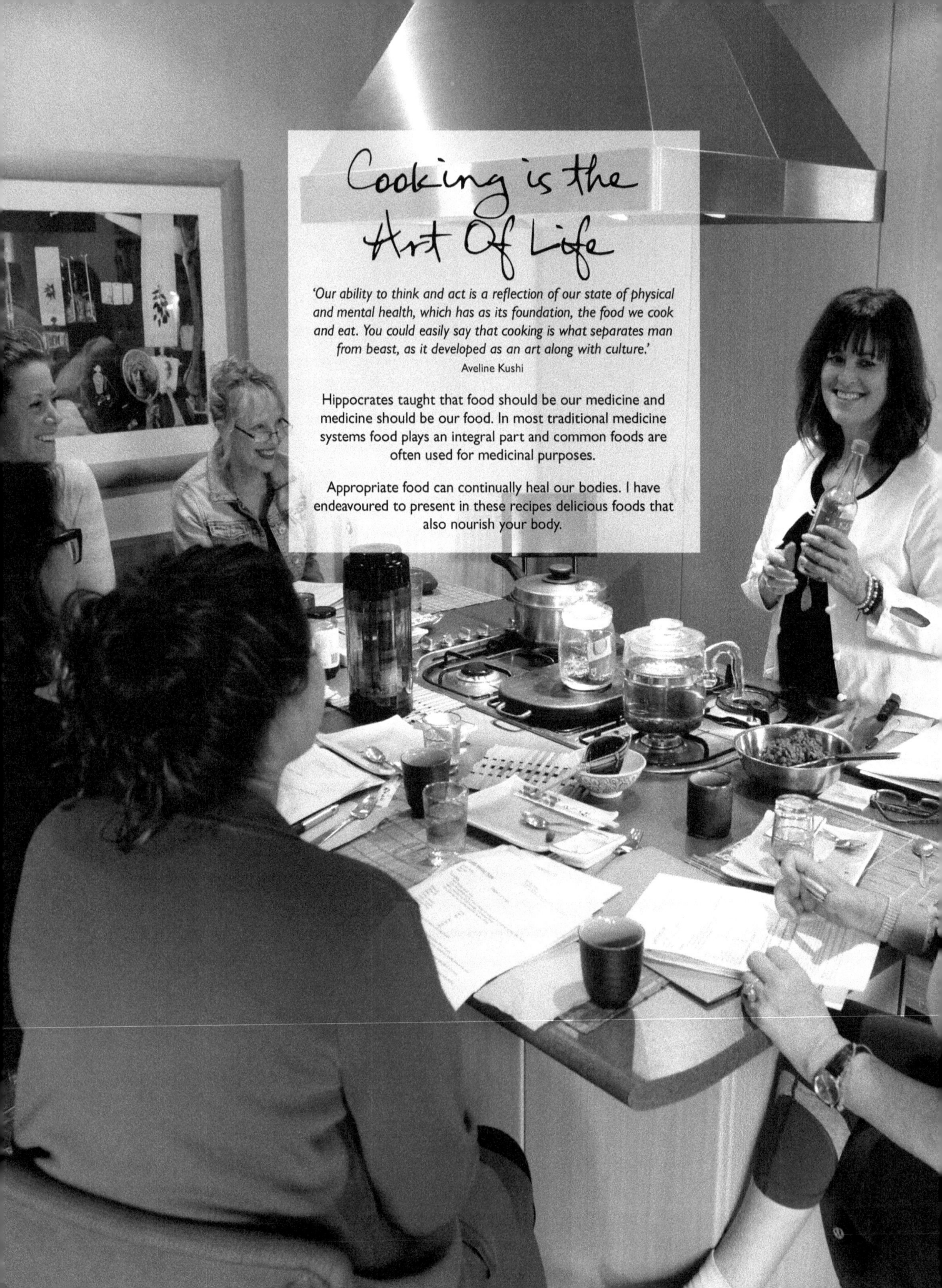

Cooking is the Art Of Life

'Our ability to think and act is a reflection of our state of physical and mental health, which has as its foundation, the food we cook and eat. You could easily say that cooking is what separates man from beast, as it developed as an art along with culture.'

Aveline Kushi

Hippocrates taught that food should be our medicine and medicine should be our food. In most traditional medicine systems food plays an integral part and common foods are often used for medicinal purposes.

Appropriate food can continually heal our bodies. I have endeavoured to present in these recipes delicious foods that also nourish your body.

Contents

My Philosophy 8

Healthy Eating Systems 9

Essential Food Groups 11

Soups - Meals In A Bowl 15

Dip : Dress : Spread : Top 35

Greens : Salads : Sea Vegetables 45

Lots More Vegetables 65

Essential Wholegrains 79

Nutritious Legumes 95

Salubrious Noodles 111

MWC Specials 123

Sweet Treats 131

My Favourite Breakfasts 147

Glossary 153

My Wholefood Journey 166

My Favourite Resources 169

Acknowledgements 170

Pantry Ingredients List 171

Index 172

Conversions 175

MY PHILOSOPHY

We all have our own unique relationship with food. I have certainly met many people with food-related issues and challenges and have heard of many 'diets' over the years.

Every day, we eat. We all have a relationship with food in some way. Some eat mindlessly, just to fill a craving and perceived hunger, some are emotional eaters. Some have health issues and are more mindful about the foods they consume. Many more do not even have food choices because of their circumstances and as there is so much poverty in the world. We have so much good food available to us in Australia and in the developed countries and we are certainly privileged to have well-researched educational resources available at our fingertips to enlighten us about good nutrition. Making the right choices just takes a little understanding and practical knowledge about how our bodies work, what are good wholefoods and what works best for us.

Many factors contribute to sickness and disease, including genetics, the environment, lifestyle and stress. Science, traditional medicine systems, anecdotal evidence and our own personal experiences inform us that we can effect positive change and prevent dis-ease by choosing wholefoods wisely. Making better food choices by eating a healthier range of plant-based wholefoods is something we can do for ourselves every meal, every day. Why feel sluggish and unwell after a day of eating the wrong foods when we have the power to feel great?

As a community, we need to become educated about what happens while we consume food: how our digestive systems work, what our organs are doing and what nutrients we are absorbing. Along with reading, writing and arithmetic, I believe this learning should form part of the school curriculum. Every child should understand how our bodies work and what nutrition supports best health. This knowledge and awareness empowers all to choose foods wisely and are preventative measures to support lifelong health.

There's more to living well than our epicurean nature might suggest. It's not just about going to the finest restaurants and drinking the best wines or the greatest coffee. One needs to maintain a daily healthy balance by choosing whole foods to provide energy, endurance, and digestive health while preventing the onset of dis-ease. (So that you know, I have a 90/10 rule: 90% plant based wholefoods and 10% treats, including coffee, chocolate and the occasional vodka.) ☺

As part of choosing wholefoods wisely we do need to pay attention to environmental factors and take the SLOW approach: choosing foods that are Seasonal, Local, Organic and Whole.
We need especially to pay attention to environmental factors. Our environment is currently cluttered with chemicals that contaminate our air, our water, our food and ourselves. What is the health effect of these environmental toxins, what is our carbon footprint, are the foods we eat genetically modified? When we look at what we eat and how we grow it, we can find evidence for damage both to our food, from pollution and soil depletion, and to our environment, from the toxicity of growing foods industrially.

The 'eat local' movement that has seen farmers markets, school garden projects and local veggie gardens flourish is an exciting backlash against the manipulation of foods. As a community we must continue to question food sources, to make growers and manufacturers accountable for the processes that food undergoes before it reaches our table. My studies and experiences all point to minimising exposure to toxins and especially to a wholefood plant-based diet being essential in providing nutrients to maintain a healthy immune system and to combat toxicity. Foods are our medicines. Drinking filtered water, eating a balanced diet of colourful fruits and vegetables, wholegrains such as brown rice and quinoa, legumes such as chickpeas and lentils, nuts and seeds, all assist in providing the essential nutrients to support your healthy body.

According to Michio and Aveline Kushi, great mentors to me:

'Cooking is the art of life. Our ability to think and act is a reflection of our state of physical and mental health, which has as its foundation the food we cook and eat. You could say cooking is what separates man from beast, as it developed as an art along with culture. To master the art of cooking – to choose the right kinds of foods and to combine them properly – is to master the art of life, for the greatness and destiny of all people reflect and are limited by the quality of their daily food. It is vitally important that you learn how to prepare food that is harmonious with your body as well as with your environment. Just as individual health is built of harmonious living and eating, so is the health and unity of the family. It is a well-known fact that highly processed foods, sugared foods and the chemicals they contain can affect behaviour and cause drastic allergic reactions in many people. The massive change in eating that has taken us from wholesome natural foods to packaged, processed, refined items has caused an equally massive decline in the health of society. Yet, a return to family orientated cooking and community living can bring health to the individual, unity and love to the family, and peace and brotherhood to society.'
(Michio Kushi, 1984 in *Changing Seasons Macrobiotic Cookbook: Cooking in Harmony with Nature* by Aveline Kushi and Wendy Esko.)

Enjoy cooking My Wholefood Community recipes and definitely enjoy eating.

Wishing you good health, naturally
Sandra

HEALTHY EATING SYSTEMS

Good nutrition maintains that the six nutrients – carbohydrates, proteins, fats, vitamins, minerals and water – are present in the foods we eat and contain chemical substances that:

- furnish the body with heat and energy
- provide material for growth and repair of body tissues
- assist in the regulation of body processes.

All the nutrients must be present in the diet in varying quantities so that the body can maintain basic life processes.

On an aeroplane to attend one of the first holistic health conferences in India in 2003, I was surprised to see on the front cover of *Newsweek International* the headline 'The Perfect Diet Beyond The Fads: What Science Tells Us about Food & Health'.

This headline on a mainstream publication was surprising and exciting.

At this holistic health conference, a gathering of the masters in the wellbeing movement, integrative medical practitioners, natural therapists, nutritionists, Ayurvedic practitioners and yoga teachers, this *Newsweek* was shared around and became a light for us all.

We read that nutrition experts from the Harvard School of Public Health created the Healthy Eating Pyramid.

It is based on the best available long term scientific evidence about the links between diet and health.

I had learnt about The Macrobiotic Healthy Eating Pyramid from Michio Kushi of the Kushi Institute Massachusetts many years ago and recently Professor Walter Willett MD., Dr. P.H. and team from the Department of Nutrition at Harvard School of Public Health used scientific research to recommend a mostly plant based diet too.

Since my discovery of the Harvard Medical School guide to healthy eating, I have shared it and the Macrobiotic Healthy Eating Pyramid with all who attend my classes and seminars. (see Macrobiotics in glossary). Note that the Macrobiotic Pyramid includes pickles, fermented foods and sea vegetables too.

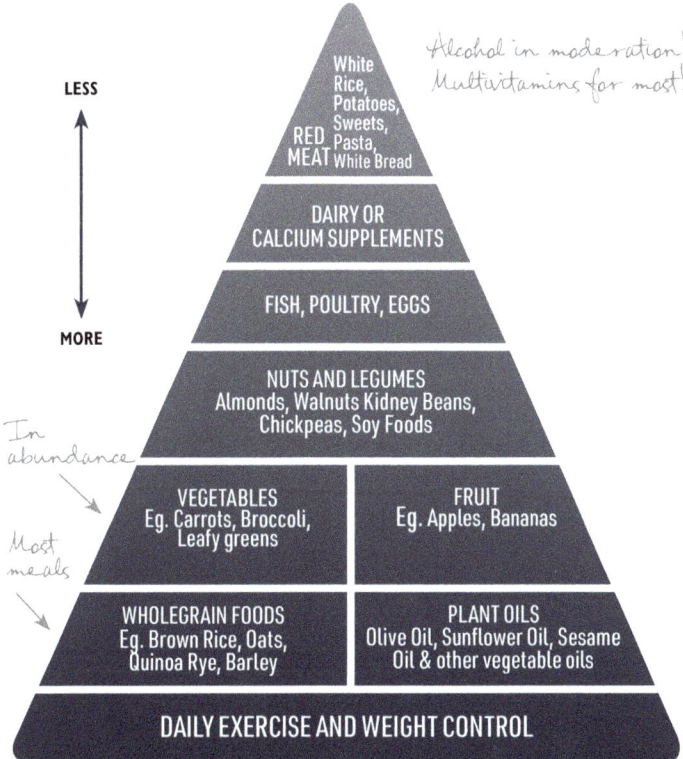

HARVARD HEALTHY EATING PYRAMID

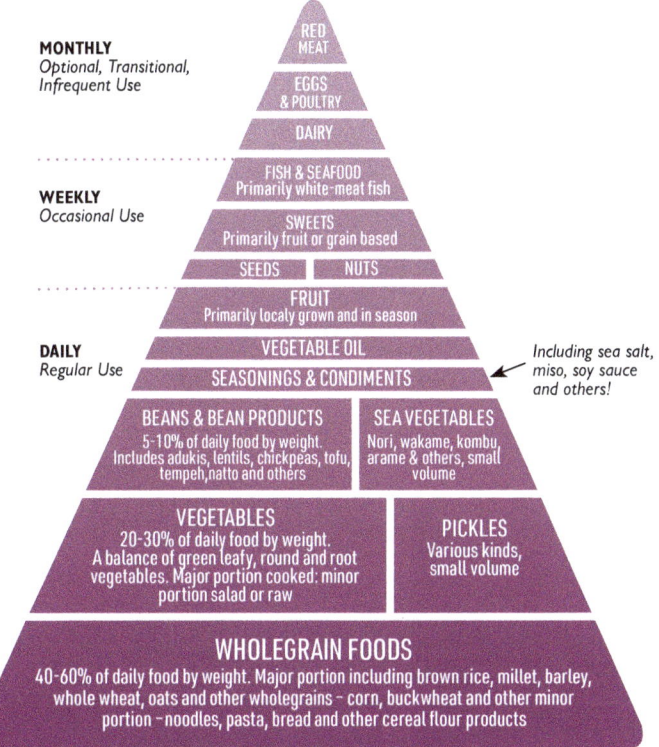

MACROBIOTIC PYRAMID

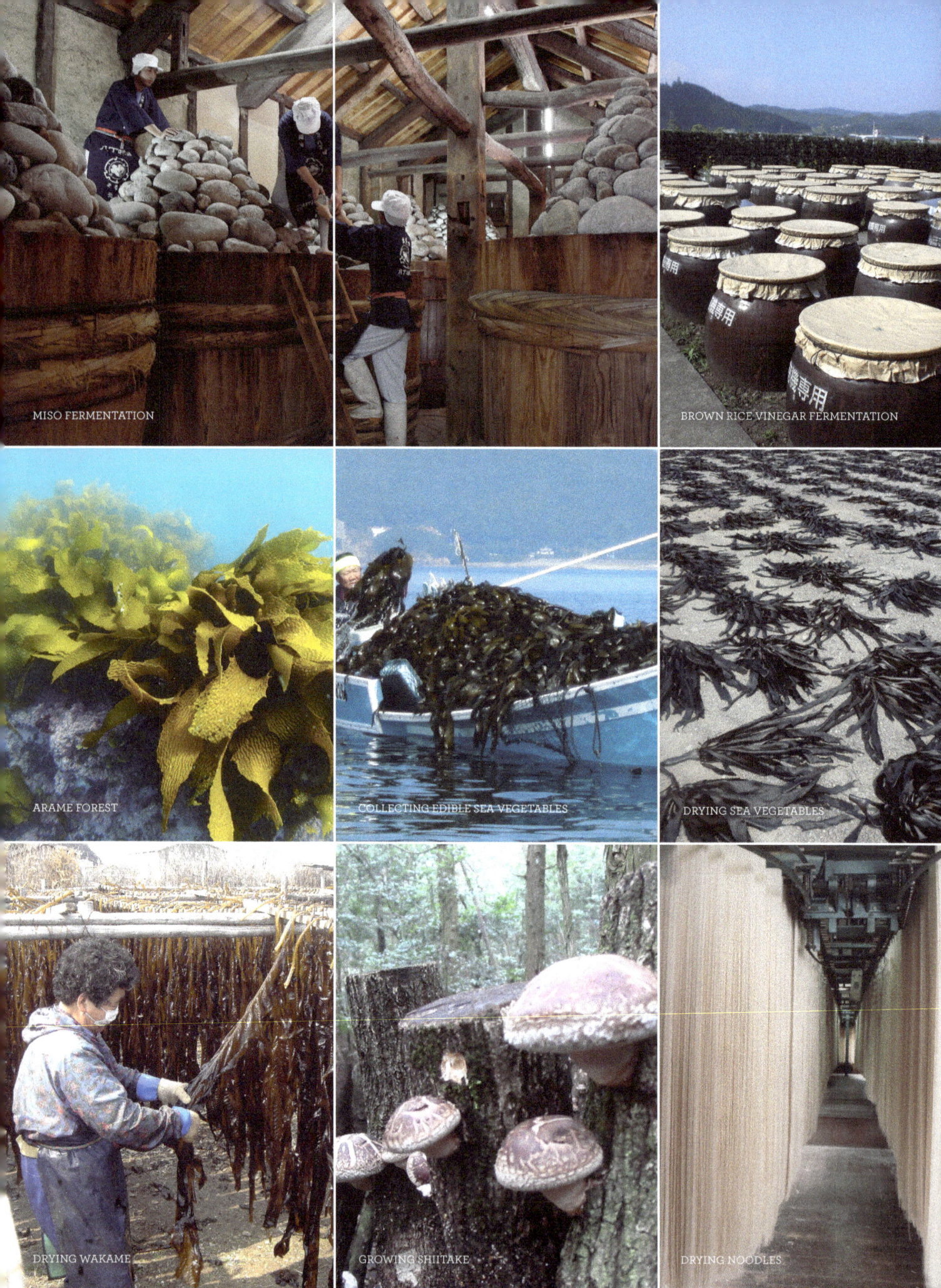

This is the health-supportive nutritional information I share with all of my wholefood community who come to any of my classes.

THE ESSENTIAL FOOD GROUPS

WHOLEGRAINS

The term 'wholegrain' is used to describe an intact grain, flour or food that contains all three parts of the grain. The intact grain or the dehulled, ground, milled, cracked or flaked grain is where the constituents – endosperm, germ and bran – are present. Together they deliver over 26 nutrients and other active substances that nourish the body and help to reduce risk of disease. Wholegrains are packed with nutrients, including protein, fibre, B vitamins, antioxidants, and trace minerals (iron, zinc, copper and magnesium).

Wholegrains provide energy and stamina, can help to calm nerves, and promote elimination, quick reflexes, good memory and clear thinking.

Examples: Brown rice, oats, millet (technically a seed), barley, wild rice, buckwheat, quinoa.

Note: Quinoa is frequently called a grain because it is used and cooked like one, and is often called an ancient grain and a wholegrain. It is, however, not a grain: it is a gluten-free super-seed. Botanically speaking, it's a relative of spinach, beets and chard. The part we eat is actually the seed.

LEGUMES/PULSES

These economical, great-tasting plant foods are low in fat, rich in fibre and protein, and have high levels of minerals such as iron, zinc, and phosphorous as well as folate and other B-vitamins.

Legumes

The term legume refers to plants whose fruit is enclosed in a pod. Well-known legumes include alfalfa, fresh peas, lupins, mesquite, soy and peanuts.

Pulses

Pulses are part of the legume family, but the term pulse refers only to the dried seed. Pulses include all beans, peas and lentils, such as baked beans; red, green, yellow and brown lentils; chickpeas (chana or garbanzo beans); garden peas; black-eyed peas; runner beans; broad beans (fava beans); adzuki beans; kidney beans; butter beans (lima beans); haricot beans (navy beans); cannellini beans; flageolet beans; pinto beans; and borlotti beans.

ABOUT PROTEIN

Good quality protein is necessary for building and repairing new tissues, transporting oxygen and nutrients in the blood and making antibodies to fight infections.

Protein occurs in all living cells and has both functional and structural properties. Protein is found throughout the body: in muscle, bone, skin, hair and virtually every other body part or tissue. Amino acids, assembled in long chains, are the building blocks of protein. Of the 20 amino acids found in proteins, some can be made by the body while others are essential in the diet. Amino acids are used for the synthesis of body proteins and other metabolites and can also be used as a source of dietary energy.

A diet focusing on plant-based protein sources (legumes, grains, nuts, seeds and vegetables from land and sea) can be beneficial in helping to prevent diabetes, cardiovascular disease and cancer and in supporting a longer healthier life. Plant proteins come packaged with fibre, carbohydrates, healthful fats and phytochemicals that protect against disease.

FYI: Wholegrains and legumes, or legumes, seeds and nuts, are complementary proteins. Complementary proteins are two or more incomplete protein sources that together provide adequate amounts of all the essential amino acids.

SEA VEGETABLES: EDIBLE SEAWEED

In my recipes I use arame, wakame, kombu, nori, dulse and agar agar.

Seaweed and marine algae have a high concentration of nutrients and they have long been considered to possess powers to prolong life, prevent disease, and impart beauty and health. For thousands of years, this mineral-rich vegetable has been a staple in Asian diets.

There are over 20 types of edible seaweed and even more are being discovered. Some types of seaweed have more calcium than cheese, more iron than beef, and more protein than eggs, plus seaweed is a very rich source of micronutrients. Traditionally, its healing properties are said to include everything from treating cancer, lowering cholesterol, shrinking goitres, dissolving tumours and cysts, detoxifying heavy metals, reducing water retention, and aiding in weight loss.

Nutrients include vitamins A, C, E, B complex and B12 as well as calcium, potassium and iron. In addition, sea vegetables are low in calories and provide protein and fibre and even some omega-3 fatty acids.

ESSENTIAL GOOD FATS

Small amounts of healthy fats, such as extra virgin olive oil, unrefined sesame oil, nuts, seeds and avocado, are needed for the proper function of the immune and hormonal systems, the manufacture of prostaglandins (which seem to play a role in the regulation and function of all organs and cells), sex hormones, cell wall construction and the transport of fat-soluble vitamins such as A, E, K and D.

Healthful fats are high in essential fatty acids (EFAs), which include omega-3 and omega-6, both associated with cardiovascular health, good skin, hair and nails, and a strong immune system. Unrefined healthful fats found in seeds and nuts contain natural antioxidants and nutrients.

A small amount of these fats can enhance the taste of a meal and also help to keep you satisfied for longer.

FYI: I use these organic oils in my recipes: extra virgin olive oil, unrefined sesame oil, toasted sesame oil, extra virgin coconut oil and organic tahini, which I also include here as it has a high oil content and is a healthy fat too.

NUTS

More is not necessarily better: eating too many nuts and seeds is not recommended. A small handful is best.

Like other plant foods, nuts provide a range of nutrients, including large quantities of healthy monounsaturated and polyunsaturated fats (49–74% total fat – except chestnuts, which are low fat), and moderate amounts of protein (9–20%).

Nuts are also a good source of fibre and provide a wide range of essential nutrients, including several B group vitamins (including folate), vitamin E, minerals such as calcium, iron, zinc, potassium and magnesium, antioxidant minerals (selenium, manganese and copper), plus other phytochemicals such as antioxidant compounds (flavonoids and resveratrol) and plant sterols.

Nuts are a well-known health food and traditional Chinese medicine (TCM) recommends nuts as part of a healthy diet, especially in winter as nuts are hot/warm yang energy foods. Eating nuts when it is cold can help reinforce energy, though eating too many nuts in warm weather can cause excessive internal heat.

Nuts are loaded with vitamins, nutrients, and unsaturated fatty acid and preliminary studies have indicated that nuts may play a role in preventing development of type 2 diabetes, reducing the risk of developing heart disease, reducing age-related macular degeneration (which can lead to blindness), maintaining bone health, slowing brain ageing and reducing cancer.

Traditional Chinese medicine (TCM) considers that nuts are especially good at reinforcing the kidney organ meridian system (the term used in TCM for kidneys and the reproductive and urinary systems). Nuts promote brain health, sharp thinking and generally build up health. Walnuts, almonds and chestnuts are especially nourishing and part of TCM dietary therapy.

All nuts are good for you but it's a good idea not to eat too many of them and to avoid salted oil-roasted nuts.

Each nut variety contains its own unique combination of nutrients. The characteristics for which each variety is particularly beneficial are listed here.

- Almonds: protein, calcium and vitamin E
- Brazil nuts: fibre and selenium (just two brazil nuts a day provide 100% RDI of selenium for an adult)
- Cashews: non-haem (plant-based) iron and low GI
- Chestnuts: low GI, fibre and vitamin C (although much vitamin C is lost during cooking)
- Hazelnuts: fibre, potassium, folate and vitamin E
- Macadamias: highest in monounsaturated fats, thiamin and manganese
- Pecans: fibre and antioxidants
- Pine nuts: vitamin E and the amino acid arginine
- Pistachios: protein, potassium, plant sterols and the antioxidant resveratrol
- Walnuts: alpha-linoleic acid, plant omega-3 and antioxidants

Nuts are naturally low in sodium, contain potassium and most contain some carbohydrate in the form of natural sugars. Chestnuts are different they are rich in low glycaemic index carbohydrates and low in fat, making them more like a grain than a tree nut.

SEEDS

Sesame and sunflower seeds are incredibly rich sources of many essential minerals. Calcium, iron, manganese, zinc, magnesium, selenium and copper are especially concentrated in seeds. Many of these minerals have a vital role in bone mineralisation, red blood cell production, enzyme synthesis and hormone production, as well as regulation of cardiac and skeletal muscle activities.

Just a handful of sesame or sunflower seeds a day provides the recommended levels of phenolic anti-oxidants, minerals, vitamins and protein.

FYI: It's best to buy organic nuts and seeds and to keep them tightly sealed in the refrigerator or freezer.

VEGETABLES AND FRUITS

Fruits and vegetables are high in fibre and contain many vitamins and minerals that are good for health. These include vitamins A (beta-carotene), C and E, magnesium, zinc, phosphorous and folic acid.

A diet rich in a variety of vegetables and fruits may lower blood pressure, reduce risk of heart disease and stroke, prevent some types of cancer, lower risk of eye and digestive problems, and have a positive effect upon blood sugar, which can help keep appetite in check.

Eat a variety of types and colours of produce in order to give your body the mix of nutrients it needs. Try dark leafy greens, brightly coloured red, yellow and orange vegetables and fruits, and cooked tomatoes.

No single fruit or vegetable provides all of the nutrients you need to be healthy. Eat plenty every day. Vegetables and fruits are an important part of a healthy diet.

CHEWING

Twenty years ago I went to study macrobiotics with Herman and Cornelia Aihara and David Briscoe in California. I was so confronted by my own lack of chewing as we spent eating time in silence and focusing just on our meal. The exercise was to chew brown rice 100 times. Initially I couldn't get past 10 chews. I did get better at chewing after about my fifth meal there and certainly it made a difference to my enjoyment of flavours and feeling completely satisfied while eating less. It did mostly become second nature to chew properly, but sometimes I still can be distracted from my meal when eating out and talking while eating with family and friends. The result is that afterwards I can't remember tasting my food and I can feel bloated and unwell.

Chewing (mastication) is the process by which food is crushed and ground by teeth. It is the first step of digestion, and it increases the surface area of foods to allow the enzymes to break the food down more efficiently. The way you chew, including how long you chew, can significantly impact your health.

The longer you chew, the more time it will take you to finish a meal, and research shows that eating slowly can help you to eat less and, ultimately, to avoid weight gain or even lose weight.

When a large particle of improperly chewed food enters your stomach, it may remain undigested when it enters your intestines. There, bacteria will begin to break it down or, in other words it will start to putrefy, potentially leading to gas and bloating, diarrhoea, constipation, abdominal pain, cramping and other digestive problems.

So now that you know, just chew your food more. The next time you take a bite, pay attention to the number of times you chew and your natural reflex to swallow. Remember digestive enzymes release in your mouth and chewing aids digestion and boosts nutrient absorption. When you consciously chew, you'll naturally slow down how quickly you're eating. When you slow down how quickly you're eating, you allow yourself the chance to be aware of your natural hunger and satiety cues, which can decrease your risk of overeating. Try chewing each bite anywhere from 15 to 30 times depending on the food. Take the time to relish and enjoy each bite. We all will be doing our whole digestive system a big favour.

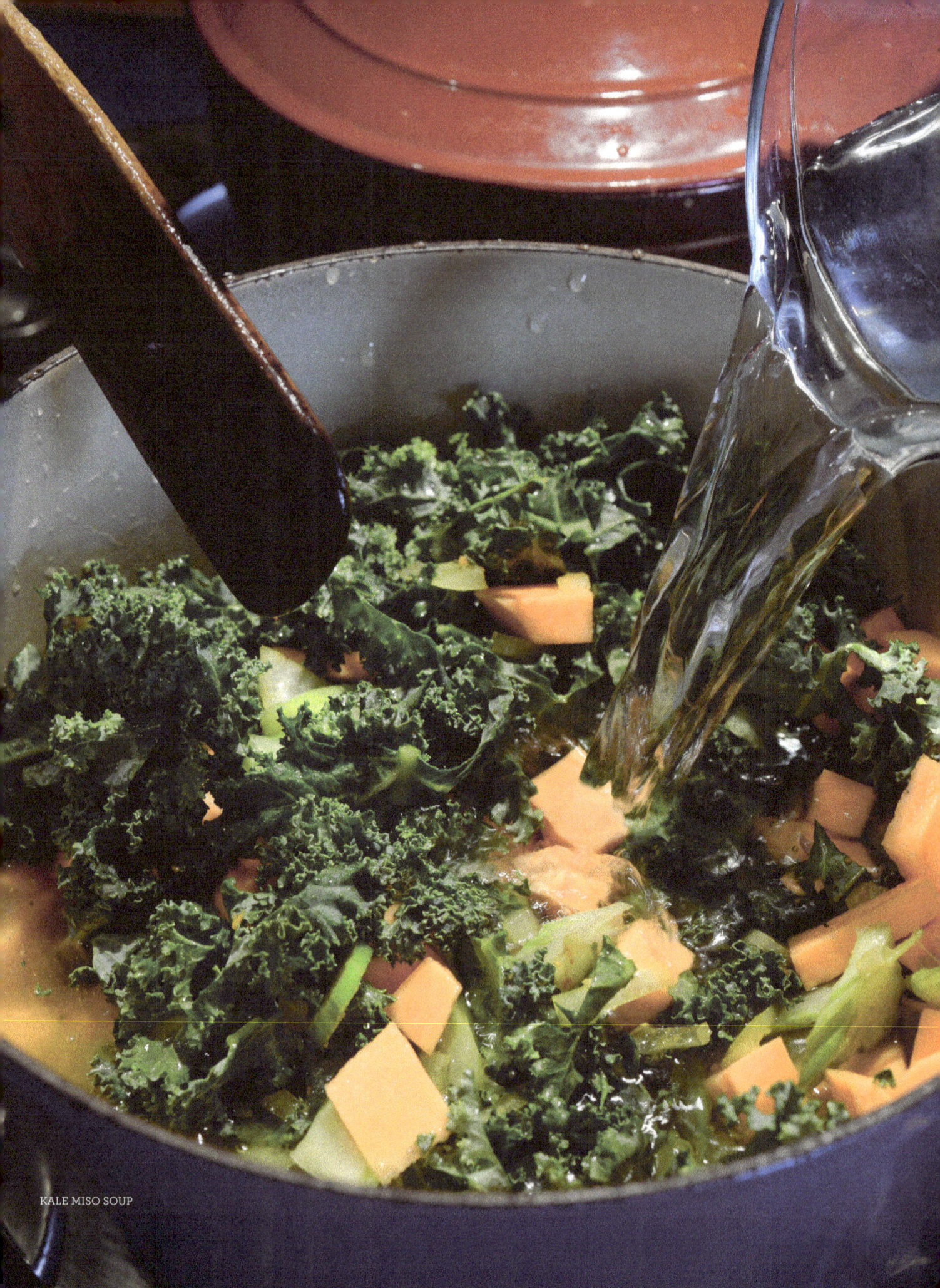

KALE MISO SOUP

Soup
[MEAL IN A BOWL]

Vegetable Stock 16

Thai Vegetable Stock 17

Tips For Cooking With Miso 19

Kale Miso Soup 19

Wakame Miso Soup 21

Broccoli Avocado Soup 22

Split Pea Soup With Smoked Tofu 25

Red Lentil Beetroot Soup 27

North African Millet Soup 29

Latin American Quinoa Bean Soup 31

Slow Cooked Spicy Black Bean & Rice Soup 33

VEGETABLE STOCK

MAKES ABOUT 2 LITRES

It doesn't matter what vegetables you use for this stock. Options are listed below:

Onions & onion peel

Greens

Carrots

Celery

Pumpkin skin

Tomatoes

Cabbage cores

Wilted lettuce or watercress

Parsley stems

Aromatics: bay leaf, rosemary, thyme, peppercorns, cumin seeds, celery seeds, coriander seeds, sage

- Place all aromatics and vegetables (including peels, skins and ends – see tip below) and a strip of wakame (kombu if you can get it) into a soup pot.
- Cover with twice as much water.
- Cover pot with lid and bring to a full boil over high heat. Reduce heat and simmer for 30 minutes to an hour.
- Strain through colander into another pot.
- Let stock cool before refrigerating.

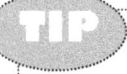

MAKING VEGETABLE STOCK

Collect peels and scraps for stock in a container. These will keep for several days in the refrigerator.

Organic vegetables are best. Wash well with a vegetable brush.

Do not use bitter or sour foods like beet greens and lemon peel, or waxed, mouldy or spoiled pieces.

Cook stock ahead of time and keep refrigerated until use. Always taste stock before using it.

The colour of the soup stock is influenced by the seasoning. A pinch of sea salt will keep the colours bright. Shoyu or tamari will darken soup.

It's always handy to keep in your pantry an organic vegetable stock, which you can buy at your health food store. If a recipe (such as the Latin American quinoa bean soup) calls for more stock than you have, just make up the difference with water.

USING HOT WATER

It is best not to use hot or warm water from the tap for cooking or drinking. Hot tap water dissolves contaminants more quickly than cold water and can taste and smell bad. Better use filtered water boiled and hot from saucepan or kettle.

THAI VEGETABLE STOCK

MAKES ABOUT 2 LITRES

2 large	Onions, quartered
4 long	Red chillies, fresh
250 g	Carrots, chopped into chunks
¼ small	White Chinese cabbage, halved
2 stalks	Celery, including leaves
50 g	Coriander, fresh, including stalks
25 g	Thai basil, fresh
1 small	Daikon radish, chopped into chunks
20	Black whole peppercorns
½ tsp	Sea salt
1 tsp	Coconut sugar
2 litres	Water (I use alkalised filtered water)

- Place all ingredients into a large heavy-based saucepan.
- Bring to a boil, cover and reduce heat to simmer for 1 hour.
- Remove cover and bring to the boil for 10 minutes.
- Allow to cool, and then strain.
- Freeze any stock you don't use straightaway.

I met Sandy way back when. I met her around the time sushi came to Australia and rice balls were the hot lunch time snack to eat. Although I had learnt lots about health from my mother, Sandy really took things to the next stage. She's an amazing person with so much to teach and she never stops helping. She has been an inspiration and a great help throughout my life with health issues I have been blessed with.

I'll never forget: Sandy invited me to help her run a cooking class. The deal was I could come for free and learn heaps on the condition I help assist her to cut food and prep. The winner... Brian Hamersfeld – I got to eat everything at the end.

We still have Sandy's nutritional information sheets and recipes from all those years ago in a bound folder. Natalie, my wife, and now our kids treasure this folder and still today cook amazing dishes from the treasure trove. I am so hungry now, I have to go eat... Sandy, where are you?

Brian Hamersfeld, Melbourne

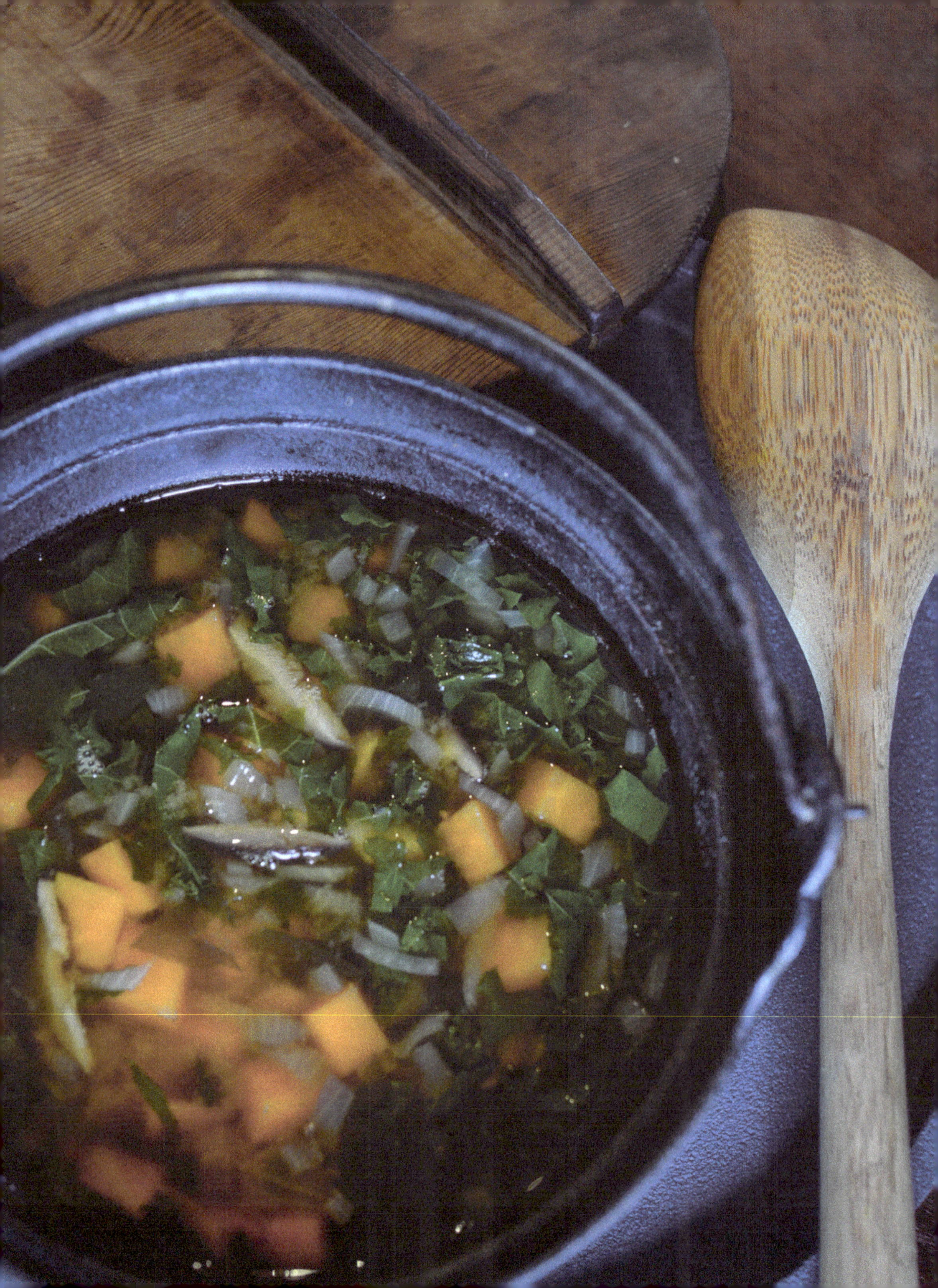

KALE MISO SOUP

FEEDS 4–6 PEOPLE
KEEPS REFRIGERATED FOR UP TO 3 DAYS

1 medium	Onion, medium diced
5	Shiitake mushrooms, dried
5 cups	Water
1 cup	Sweet potato, medium diced
2 cups	Kale, chopped
8 cm	Wakame, dried
1 tbsp	Sesame or coconut oil
3 tbsp	Miso paste (I prefer dark miso paste like Hatcho, Mugi or Genmai)
To taste	Ginger juice (grate ginger then squeeze to release juice)
1	Spring onion, chopped for garnish

I prefer the flavour of dried Japanese shiitake mushrooms — (see picture in glossary p.161)

- Soak shiitake mushrooms for at least 30 minutes in 5 cups warm water from the kettle (see tip p.16) or for even better flavour, soak overnight.
- When mushrooms have softened, discard stems then slice mushrooms caps. Strain shiitake soaking water and keep as soup stock.
- Soak wakame in enough water to cover until soft (approx. 10 minutes), remove stem and chop. Retain soaking water to add to soup. (I toss the stems onto my vegie garden as fertiliser.)
- In a soup pot, sauté diced onion in oil until transparent. Mix in sliced shiitake.
- Add the 5 cups of strained shiitake soaking water, bring to boil, then reduce heat to simmer for 5 minutes. You can add any strained wakame soaking water at this point too.
- Add sweet potato and kale to soup then simmer for about 10 minutes more (until veggies are cooked).
- Add chopped wakame and simmer 2 minutes.
- Remove soup from heat.
- Remove 1 cup soup, pour into a jug and add miso paste. Once the miso has dissolved, return liquid to pot and wait for a couple of minutes before serving.
- Add ginger juice to your taste.
- Garnish with chopped spring onions

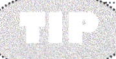

COOKING WITH MISO

For all information about miso, including pictures of the manufacturing process, see the glossary.

Do not boil miso!

Miso doesn't dissolve well when you add it directly to a soup. Because of this, I always recommend dissolving in a separate bowl or jug, either using liquid from the soup or additional water.

If you make a big pot of any of my miso soups to enjoy over a couple of days, my tip is to store them without the miso. Then, when heating your portion, add a little miso paste to your soup bowl, then ladle on hot soup to mix in the bowl. This keeps naturally fermented miso active.

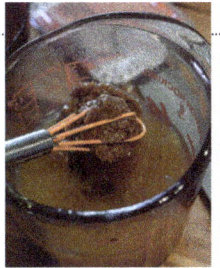
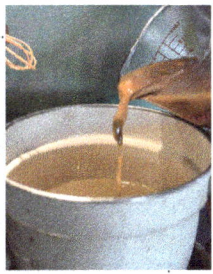

Some recipes specify the type of miso to use, others simply call for miso paste. Where I haven't specified a type, you're free to choose your own. Light miso pastes, such as Shiro, are sweeter and less salty than dark miso pastes, such as Genmai and Mugi, which have a more intense flavour.

If using miso paste, use about 1 tbsp paste for 2 cups liquid.

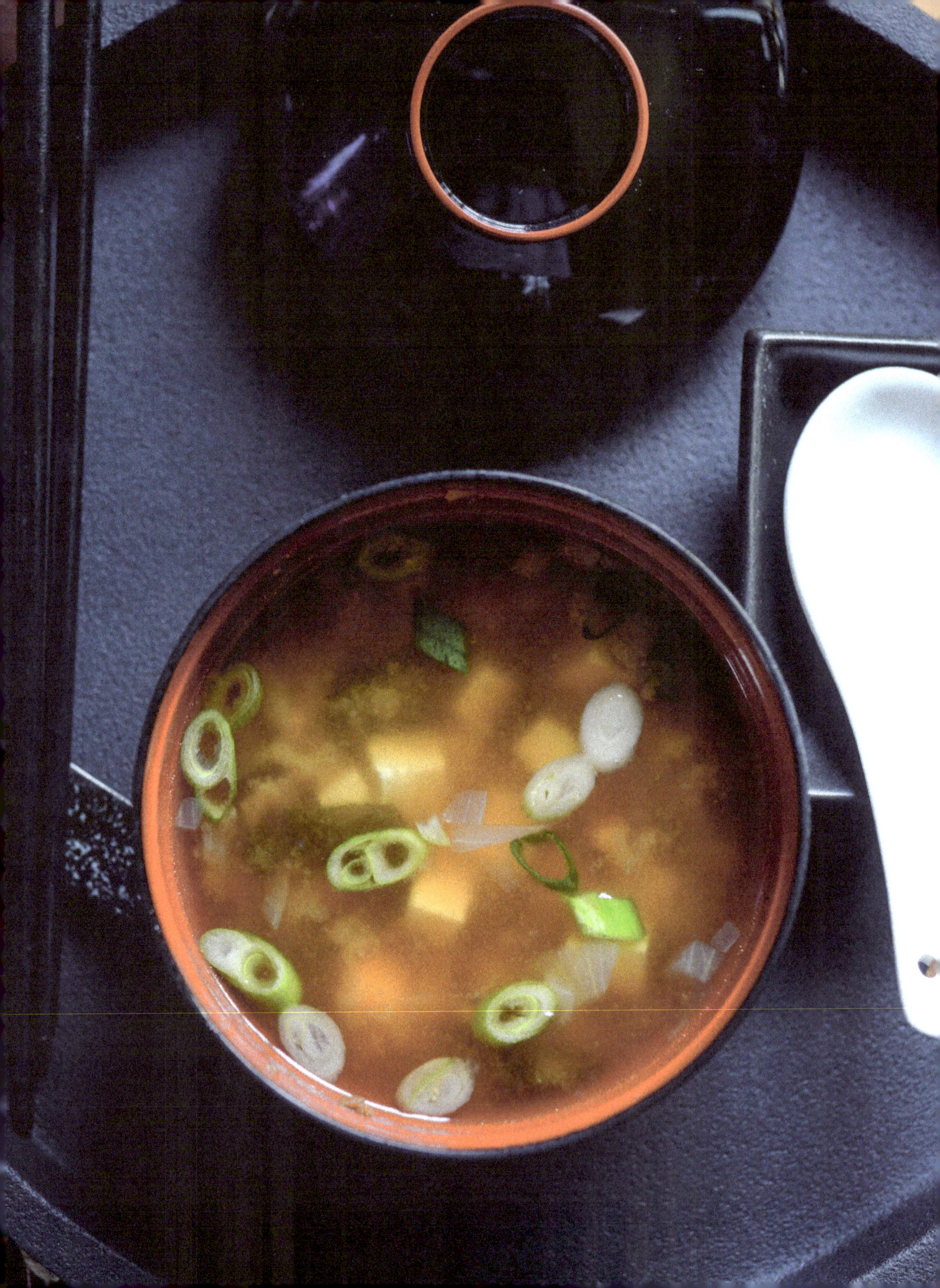

WAKAME MISO SOUP

EASILY FEEDS 4 PEOPLE
KEEPS REFRIGERATED FOR UP TO 3 DAYS

1 tbsp	Sesame oil
1 medium	Onion, diced (use fennel if you don't like onions)
1 medium	Carrot, diced
4	Shiitake mushrooms, dried
8 cm	Wakame sea vegetable, dried
5 cups	Water
4–5 tbsp	Dark miso paste (Genmai or Mugi are best)
1	Spring onion, chopped
100–200 g	Tofu, firm

I can see in my large recipe file that I have been sharing this recipe since 1987!

- Soak shiitake mushrooms for at least 30 minutes in 5 cups warm water from the kettle or for even better flavour, soak overnight.
- When mushrooms have softened, discard stems then slice mushrooms caps. Strain shiitake soaking water and keep to use as soup stock.
- Soak wakame in enough water to cover until soft (approx. 10 minutes), remove stem and chop. Retain soaking water to add to soup.
- Place block of tofu in a bowl and pour boiling water over it. Allow it to steep for 5 minutes then drain and cut into cubes. (See Tofu in glossary.)
- In a soup pot, heat sesame oil then add onion (or fennel, if using) and sauté until transparent. Add diced carrot and sliced shiitakes.
- Add the strained shiitake soaking water (about 5 cups) and bring to the boil. Then reduce heat and simmer for 10 minutes.
- Add chopped wakame plus strained wakame soaking water. Simmer for 5 minutes more.
- Remove soup from heat.
- Remove 1 cup soup, pour into a jug and mix in miso paste. Once the miso has dissolved, return liquid to pot and wait for a couple of minutes before serving.
- Garnish with chopped spring onions and cubed tofu.

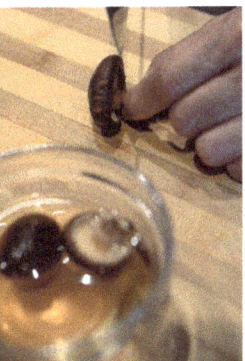 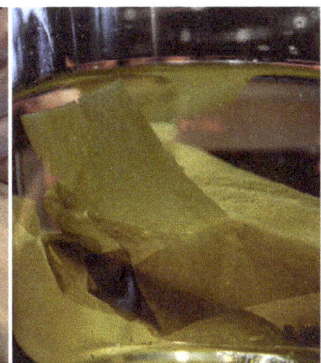 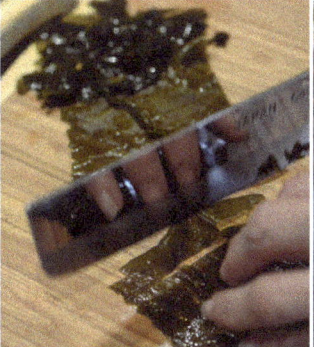 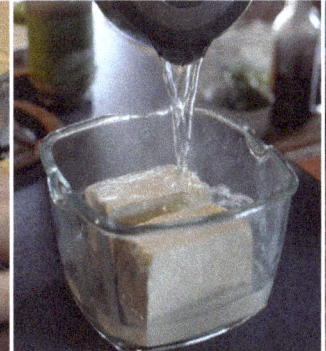 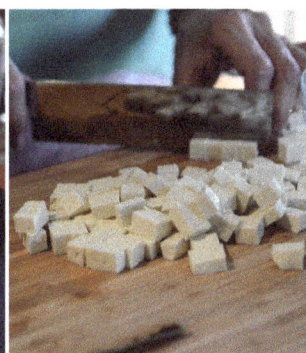

BROCCOLI AVOCADO SOUP

SERVES 2 OR 3
KEEP REFRIGERATED. BEST USED WITHIN 2 DAYS

8 florets	Broccoli
3 cups	Water
½	Avocado
½	Red onion, roughly chopped (or use fennel instead)
1 stalk	Celery, roughly chopped
Handful	Spinach leaves (or kale)
3 cm	Wakame sea vegetable, dried
1 tsp	Ginger, grated
1 large	Garlic clove, minced
1 tsp	Cumin, ground
2 tbsp	Miso paste
½ tsp	Black pepper, ground
Garnish	Roasted almond pieces
Optional	Lemon juice
Optional	Chilli pepper

- Wash broccoli, celery and spinach leaves very well.
- Soak wakame in enough water to cover until soft (approx. 10 minutes), remove stem and chop. Add strained soaking water to blender.
- Lightly steam broccoli (in a bamboo steamer is best) over a pot filled with 3 cups water for 5 to 6 minutes, until softened. Keep steaming water.
- Place steamed broccoli in blender with the rest of ingredients (except garnish and optional ingredients).
- Add steaming water as required. For a thicker, sauce-like consistency, use less water (this sauce is tasty on noodles and steamed vegetables).
- Serve with roasted almond pieces and, if desired, a few extra pieces of avocado, some chilli pepper and a splash of lemon juice.

The vegetables, wakame and miso combine to make this a nutritious soup, ideal to counter the quantity of acid-forming foods we tend to eat and to help restore our body to a healthier pH balance. In addition, the miso provides healthy bacteria that can help create the ideal environment in our digestive systems. The ingredients combine to create an amazing mix of vitamins and minerals. You can store leftover soup in the refrigerator for 2 days.
Try a miso soup once or twice a day for 10 days and see how you feel.

This is a big favourite!
It's super tasty and quick to make. It also works well as a sauce.

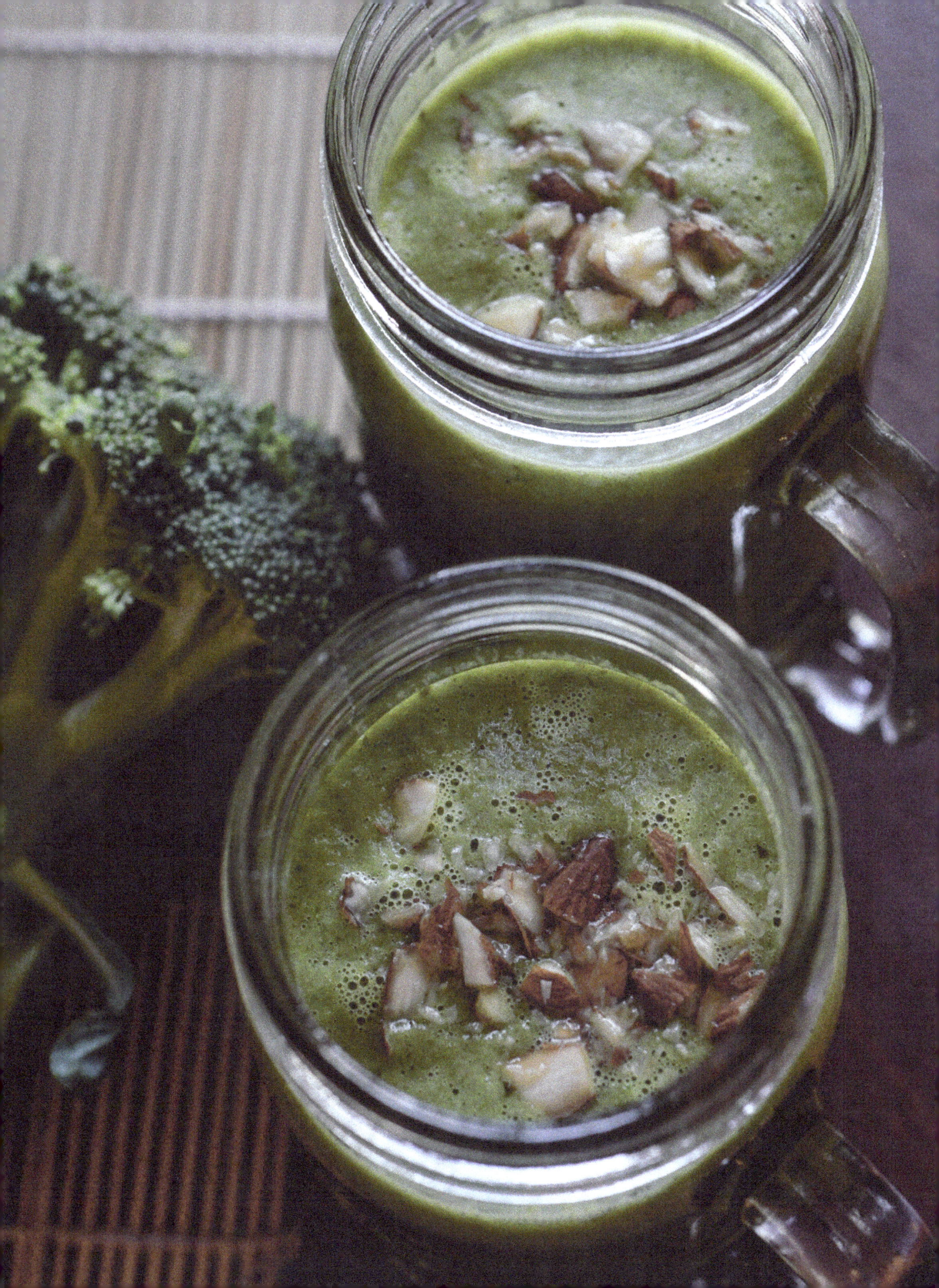

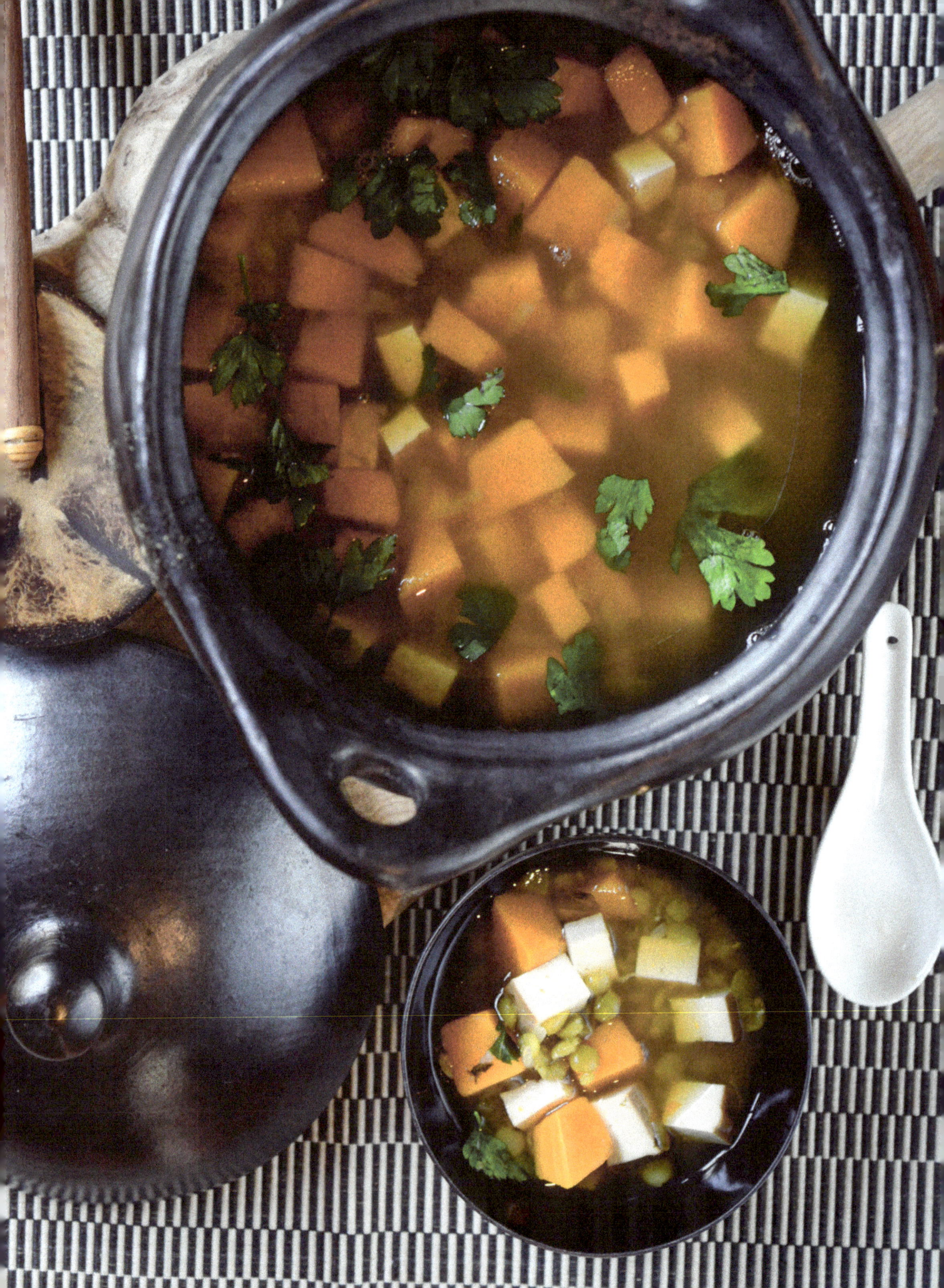

SPLIT PEA SOUP WITH SMOKED TOFU

SERVES 4
KEEP REFRIGERATED. BEST USED WITHIN 2 DAYS

1 cup	Green split peas
5 cups	Water
1 cup	Pumpkin, 3 cm diced (you can keep skin if not too thick)
½ cup	Onion, diced
5 cm	Wakame sea vegetable
To taste	Miso paste or tamari or shoyu
Garnish	Parsley, chopped

- Soak wakame in enough water to cover until soft (approx. 10 minutes), remove stem and chop. Add strained soaking water to soup.
- Wash green split peas well.
- Bring water to boil, add peas and skim off froth as needed. When the top of the water is quite clear of froth, cover pot and turn down heat to a low simmer.
- Allow peas about 30 minutes to cook. When almost done, add diced pumpkin, onions and chopped wakame, cover and cook for a further 15 minutes on low simmer.
- Blend the soup to your liking – you can blend some of the soup and keep some of it chunky, or blend it all, or not blend any.
- When vegetables are tender, add diced smoked tofu.
- Season with miso paste (dissolve in a little removed soup stock first), or tamari or shoyu.
- Garnish to serve.

I first met Sandra (Dubsy) through her work at the National Institute of Integrative Medicine (NIIM) and Professor Avni Sali, who champions complementary medicine and self-help for people with serious health challenges. Having never cooked and needing to learn how to quickly, my youngest son and I decided to attend a series of Sandra's classes and a Japanese cooking demonstration, which was particularly enthralling. Sandra's passion and enthusiasm for whole foods seemed to me the best and most sensible way to approach cooking by using natural and organic produce and her approach appealed to me. The few cooking attempts since have been complete failures, but that is no reflection on Sandra's teaching, just my ability.

David Bardas, Melbourne

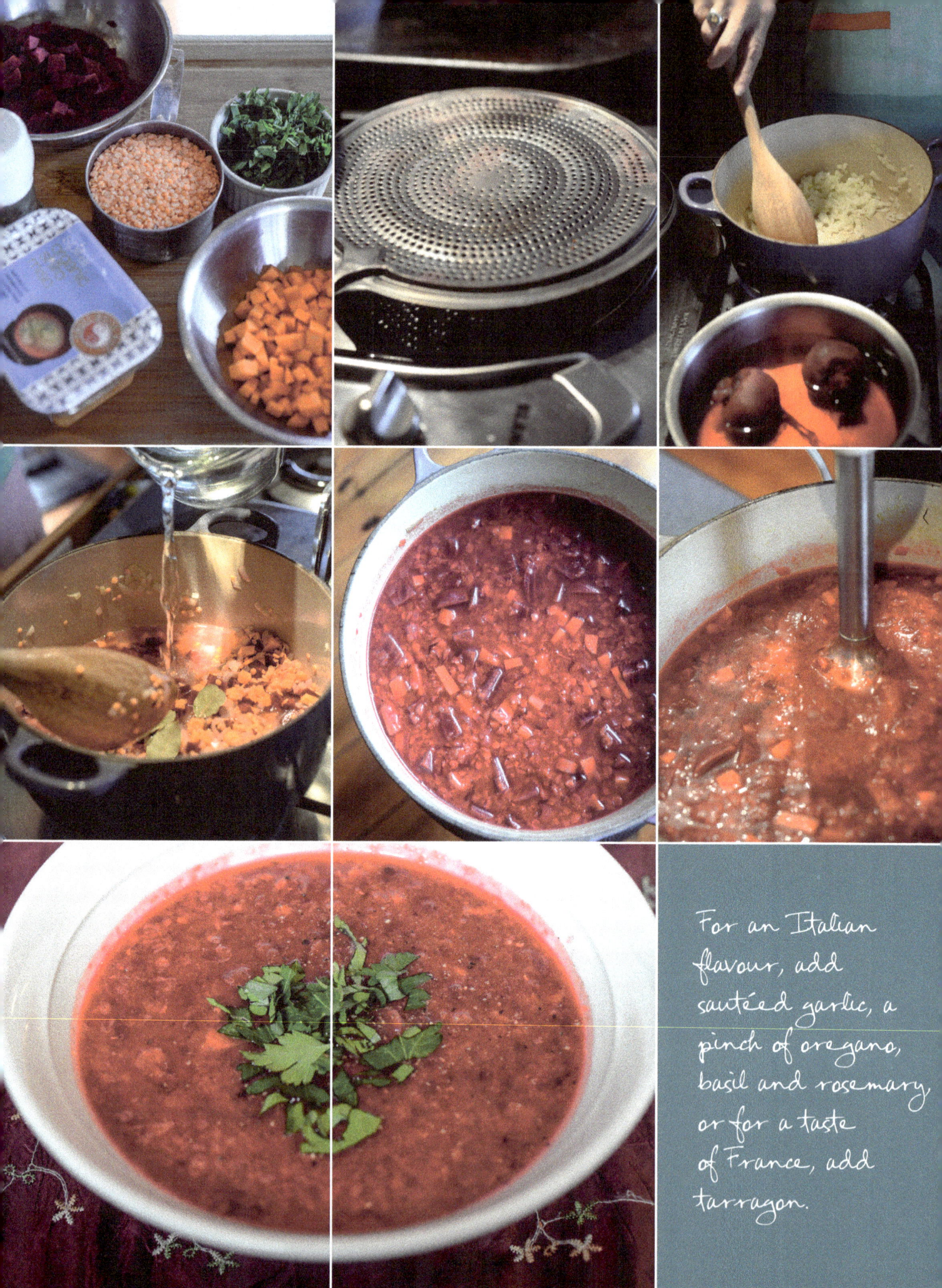

For an Italian flavour, add sautéed garlic, a pinch of oregano, basil and rosemary or for a taste of France, add tarragon.

RED LENTIL BEETROOT SOUP

SERVES 4–6 BIG BOWLS
KEEPS REFRIGERATED FOR UP TO 3 DAYS

1 tbsp	Sesame oil
1 large	Onion, medium diced
1 cup	Red lentils
2 medium	Carrots, chopped
2 large	Beetroot, peeled and chopped
5 cups	Water
8 cm	Wakame sea vegetable, dried
3	Bay leaves
3 tbsp	Miso paste (I like using Genmai miso)
To taste	Black pepper, ground
Garnish	Parsley, chopped
1–2 tsp	Plum vinegar (I use Spiral Foods Plum Vinegar – Ume Su)

- Soak wakame in enough water to cover until soft (approx. 10 minutes), remove stem and chop. Retain soaking water to add to soup.
- Wash and drain red lentils.
- Heat oil in a large soup pot and sauté onion for 5 minutes, stirring with wooden spoon.
- Add lentils, carrots, beetroots, water, chopped wakame and bay leaves then bring slowly to boil.
- Reduce heat (use a flame diffuser if you have one) and simmer for 40 to 45 minutes, or until lentils and vegetables are softened. Turn off heat.
- Remove bay leaves and discard.
- Puree in a blender or food processor then return to pot. You can leave it a bit chunky if you like. (I often use my stick blender and I'm really careful with not scratching good saucepans.)
- Dissolve miso paste in ½ cup water then mix into soup. You can also add a little miso paste to individual soup bowls if desired.
- If the soup is too thick for you, add more water.
- When serving, sprinkle with black pepper and garnish with chopped parsley and a dash of plum vinegar (Ume Su).

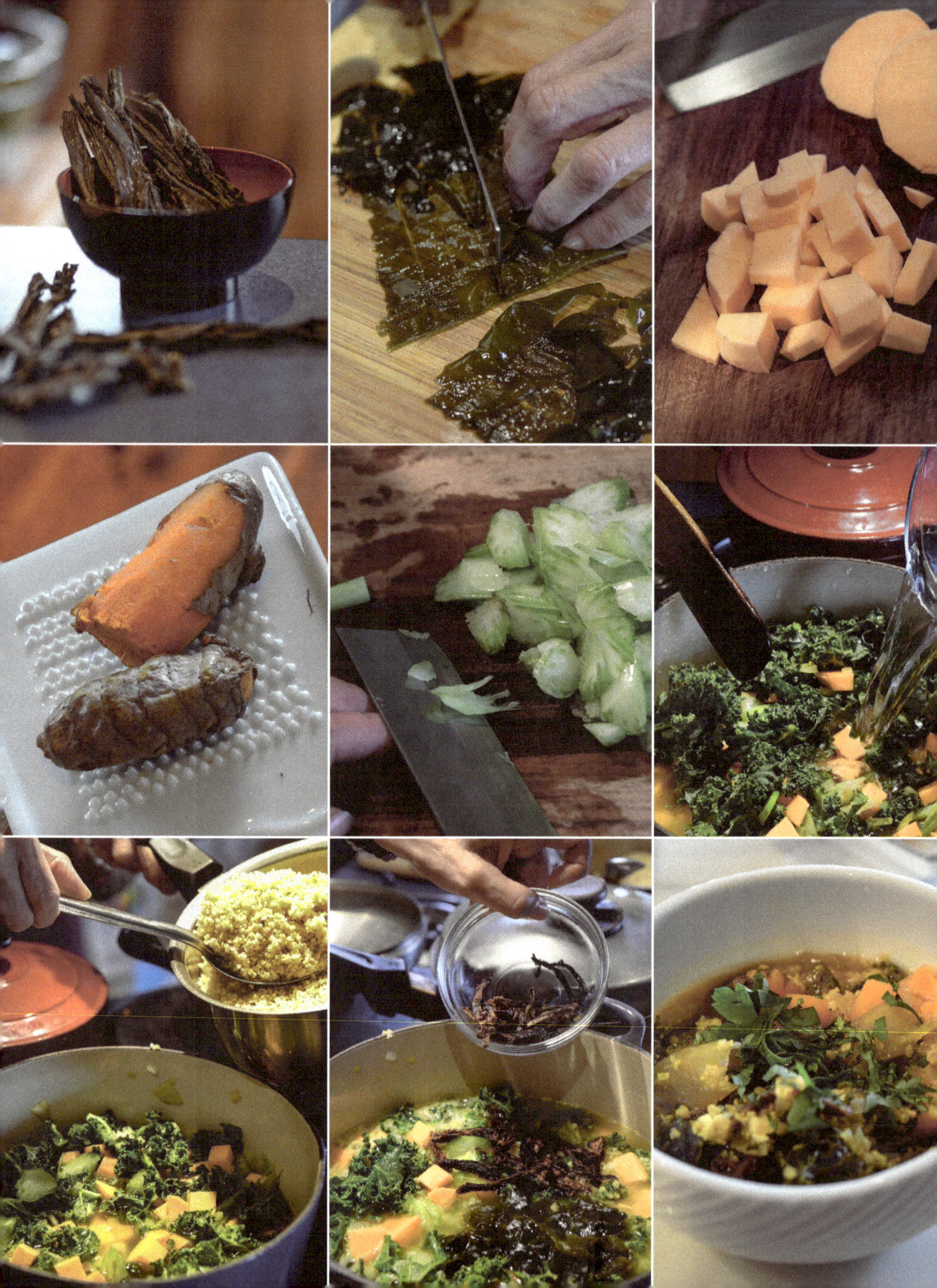

NORTH AFRICAN MILLET SOUP

MAKES 4–5 LARGE BOWLS
KEEPS REFRIGERATED FOR UP TO 3 DAYS

1–2 cups	Hulled millet, cooked (see recipe)
1 tbsp	Extra virgin olive oil
1 medium	Onion, diced
2 tsp	Ground cumin
2 tsp	Turmeric, fresh grated or 1 tsp powder
1 stalk	Celery, sliced on diagonal
2 cups	Kale, chopped
2 cups	Pumpkin or sweet potato, chopped into bite-sized cubes, about 2–3cm
5 cups	Water
½ cup	Sun-dried tomatoes (not oily), sliced into strips
10 cm	Wakame sea vegetable, dried
2–3 cloves	Garlic
2–3 tbsp	Dark miso paste (I prefer Genmai or Mugi miso)
Garnish	Parsley, fresh chopped

- Soak wakame in enough water to cover until soft (approx. 10 minutes), remove stem and chop. Retain soaking water to add to soup.
- In a large soup pot, heat oil, add diced onions and sauté with wooden spoon for 2 minutes. Add cumin and turmeric and sauté for 1 minute.
- Stir in sliced celery, chopped kale, cubed pumpkin or sweet potato and water (including wakame soaking water).
- Add cooked millet (you decide how much), sliced sun-dried tomatoes and chopped wakame and bring to a boil, then reduce heat, cover and simmer for 10 minutes.
- Squeeze garlic through a garlic press into the soup. Simmer for 5 minutes and remove from heat.
- Remove 2 cups soup, pour into a jug and add miso paste. Once the miso has dissolved, return liquid to pot.
- Serve, garnishing with chopped parsley.

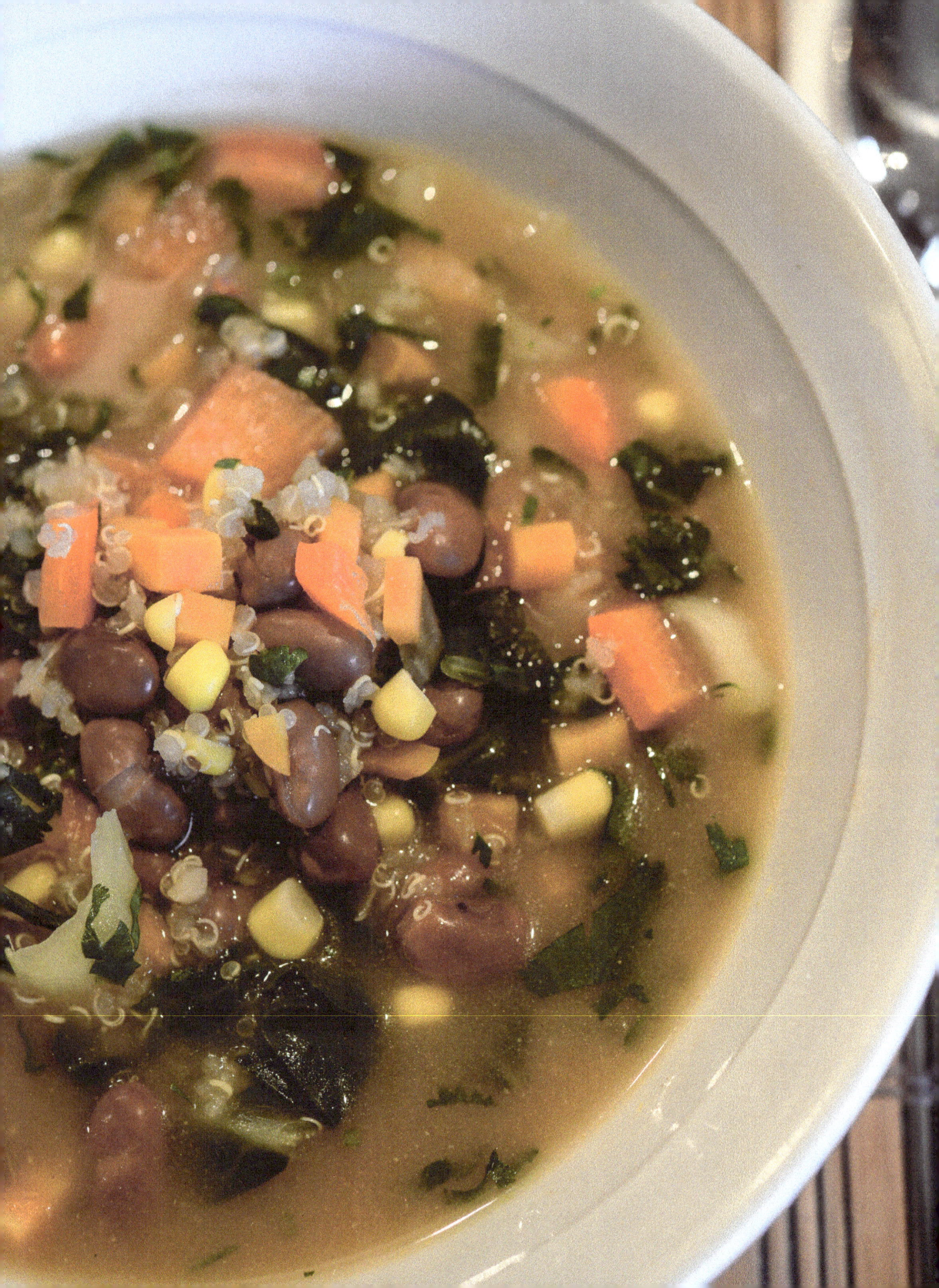

LATIN AMERICAN QUINOA BEAN SOUP

FEEDS 4–6 PEOPLE
KEEPS REFRIGERATED FOR UP TO 3 DAYS

1 tbsp	Extra virgin olive oil
1 tbsp	Garlic, minced
2 tsp	Cumin seeds or powder
6 cups	Vegetable stock (see recipe p.16)
1 large	Carrot, medium diced
1 cup	Corn kernels, fresh
¼ tsp	Cayenne pepper
1 tsp	Sea salt
400 g	Pinto beans, dried, cooked or tinned
2 cups	Greens, chopped (e.g. bok choy, kale, beet leaves)
½ cup	Red capsicum, large diced
½ cup	Quinoa, uncooked
½ cup	Coriander or parsley, fresh, finely chopped for garnish
1–2 tbsp	Lime juice
3 tbsp	White miso paste, optional (Shiro is preferred here)

- If using dried beans, soak overnight or all day first. Rinse.
- Rinse quinoa well.
- In a large soup pot, heat oil then add minced garlic and cumin and stir frequently for 2 minutes.
- Add stock and bring to the boil. Add carrot, soaked dried beans (if using), corn kernels, cayenne pepper and sea salt and return to the boil for a couple of minutes.
- Lower heat, cover and simmer for 30 minutes if using dried beans. If using tinned beans (added next), only simmer for 10 minutes.
- Add tinned beans (if using), chopped greens, capsicum and quinoa, and continue to simmer until quinoa is cooked and beans are heated – about 15 minutes.
- Remove from heat.
- For bonus nutritious flavour, remove 1 cup soup, pour into a jug and add miso paste. Once the miso has dissolved, return liquid to pot.
- Before serving, stir in chopped coriander or parsley and lime juice.

NOTE: *If you use tinned beans, this recipe will take less time.*

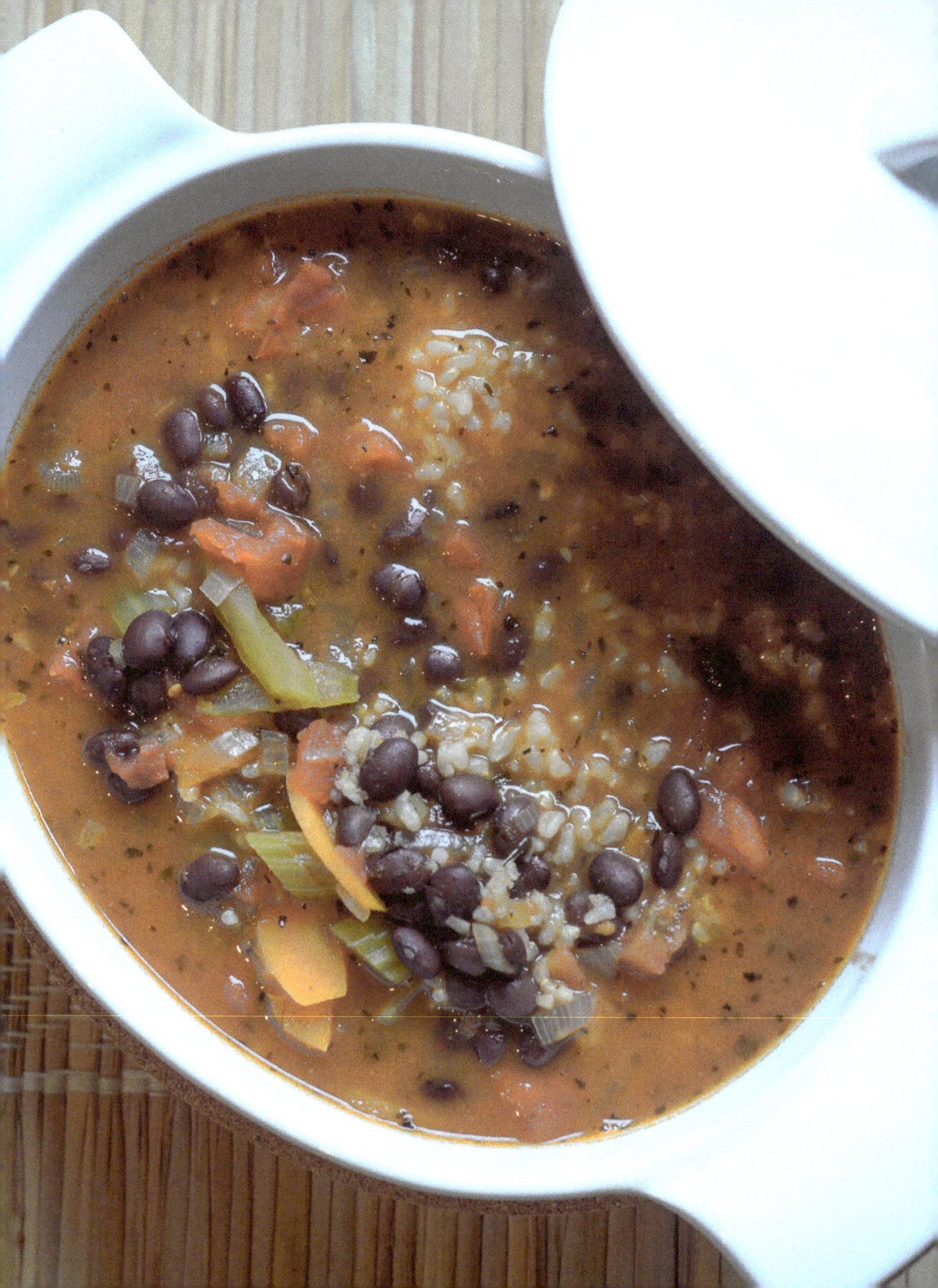

SLOW COOKED SPICY BLACK BEAN & RICE SOUP

FEEDS 4–6

1 medium	Onion, chopped
1 large	Carrot, thinly sliced
1 stalk	Celery, thinly sliced
2–3 cloves	Garlic, minced
1 tsp	Cumin, ground
1 tsp	Basil, dried
1 tsp	Chilli powder or chilli sauce
½ tsp	Oregano, dried
400 g tin	Black beans, drained and rinsed
400 g tin	Crushed tomatoes
2 cups	Vegetable stock (see recipe)
1–2 cups	Cooked brown rice (see recipe)

I hope you have homemade organic vegetable stock in your refrigerator or freezer. Get ready to use it.
If not then make it first or, even though homemade is best, you can buy it ready made in your health food store.

- Add all ingredients except rice to slow cooker.
- Cover and cook on low for 8 to 10 hours (or on high for 3 to 4 hours).
- Once soup is done, add cooked brown rice and stir to combine.
- Adjust seasonings to serve.

Instead of black beans you can use kidney beans, chickpeas or cannellini beans.

TIP

SLOW COOKER

The slow cooker, sometimes known as a crock pot, is one of the best time-saving appliances in the kitchen. It's great for beginner cooks because all you have to do is fill it and turn it on.
Hours later, you come home to a house filled with wonderful smells and dinner ready.

Soups and stews are probably the best recipes to cook in your slow cooker. Just about any soup recipe you have in your collection will work in the slow cooker with very little adjustment. You might want to reduce the liquid in a regular recipe by about one quarter to one third, simply because in your slow cooker there's no evaporation and foods actually give off liquid as they cook. If you use the same amount of liquid in your slow cooker as in the regular recipe, the soup or stew may be too diluted.

Slow cooking benefits your health and your wallet since it simplifies cooking economical and protein-rich bean dishes that typically take a long time to prepare.

The more complex and compelling flavours of slow-cooked meals are due to the extended, gentle cooking style. Cooking this way allows the flavours of the ingredients to be fully released and to blend together for delicious full-bodied flavour.

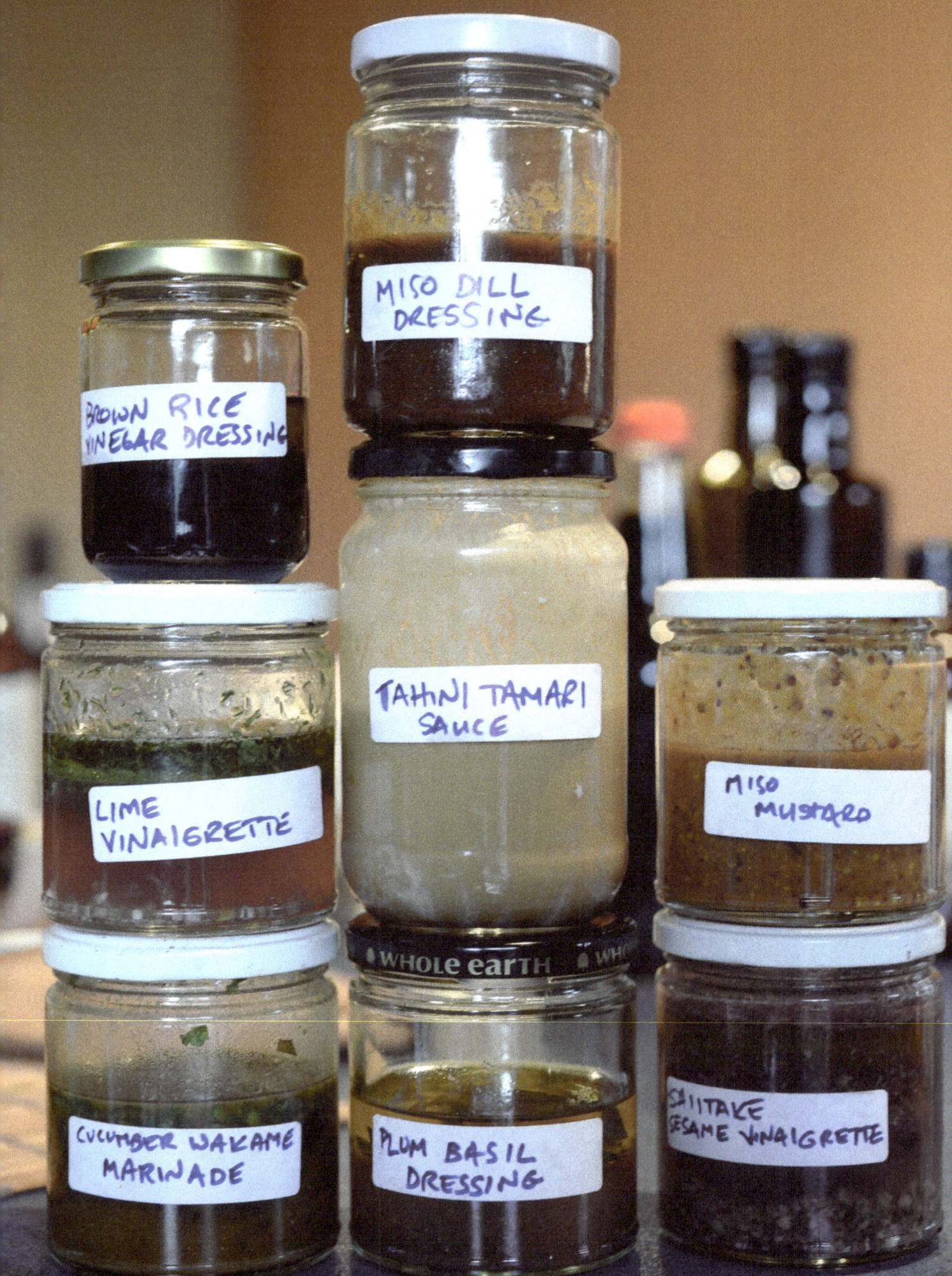

One of the secrets of delicious vegetarian food

Dip : Dress : Spread : Top

Lentil Walnut Paté 36	**IN RECIPES:**
Miso Tahini Lemon Sauce 36	Ume Tahini Dressing [Naturally Pickled Pressed Salad] 47
Miso Umeboshi Sauce 38	Plum Basil Dressing [Spring Salad] 52
Green Miso Pesto 382	Sesame Dressing [Spinach Roll – Horenso No Goma-Ae] 55
Tofu Beetroot Dip 39	Creamy Ginger Dressing [Simply Boiled Kale] 57
Chickpea Celery Hummus 40	Cucumber Wakame Salad Marinade 57
Tex-Mex Pinto Bean Dip 40	Sweet Tahini Apple Cider Dressing [Baked Beetroot, Grilled Snake Bean & Fennel] 69
Raw Beetroot Avocado Spread 41	
Adzuki Bean Spread 41	White Miso Sauce [Vegetable Noodle (Voodle) Stir Fry] 71
Miso Dill Dressing 42	
Lime Vinaigrette 42	Cashew 'Cheese' Sauce [Baked Vegetable Noodles (Voodles)] 73
Shiitake Sesame Vinaigrette 42	Tofu Sour Cream [Zucchini Pancakes] 75
Red Curry Paste 43	Miso mustard [Quinoa corn arame salad] 91
Almond Satay Sauce 43	
Miso Teriyaki Paste 43	

Use a spoon or spread with a knife for these – double-dipping can transfer bacteria from mouth to dip.

LENTIL WALNUT PATÉ

KEEPS REFRIGERATED FOR UP TO 5 DAYS

Dried lentils are a year-round staple in my pantry, essential for rounding out salads during hot weather and hearty soups in the winter months.

Buy the freshest organic dried lentils you can find and then use them within a few months. Best to store in glass jars in a cool location. Older lentils take longer to cook and tend to shed their skins during cooking.

¾ cup	Dried green or brown lentils
1	Bay leaf
1 cup	Walnuts, raw
1 tbsp	Extra virgin olive oil
1 medium	Onion, finely chopped
1 tbsp	Garlic, minced
1 tbsp	Mirin
1 tbsp	Umeboshi paste
2 tbsp	White miso paste (Shiro)
1 tbsp	Basil, dried
½ tsp	Ground black pepper
1	Spring onion, garnish
To serve	Lettuce cups (I like iceberg or witlof)

Eat this delicious paté on steamed veggies.

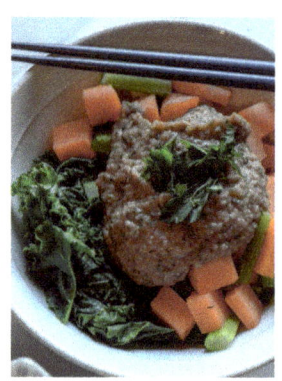

- Place lentils into a strainer. Remove any stones and rinse lentils very well under running water.
- Place lentils into a medium-sized heavy-based pot, add bay leaf and pour in enough water to cover lentils by 3 cm.
- Bring to boil over medium-high heat, then reduce heat to simmer, and cook partially covered with saucepan lid for 20 to 30 minutes, until lentils are tender but not overcooked.
- Strain and keep any remaining liquid to add to paté if required.
- Discard bay leaf. Allow lentils to cool before adding to food processor.
- Heat oven to 120°C and toast raw walnuts for about 6 minutes. Cool, then roughly chop before adding to food processor.
- Heat the olive oil in a heavy-based frypan. Sauté the onion and garlic until slightly browned, about 5 minutes. Stir in the mirin. Allow to cool before adding to food processor.
- Add the umeboshi paste, miso, basil and black pepper to the food processor and puree. Add reserved lentil cooking liquid if required for a smoother consistency.
- Serve in small scoops on lettuce cups garnished with thin slivers of spring onion.

MISO TAHINI LEMON SAUCE
A great topping for Millet Cauliflower Mash,
brown rice, noodles, patties, pancakes and crackers

MAKES ABOUT ½ CUP OR MORE IF YOU ADD MORE WATER

2 tbsp	Miso paste (your choice)
3 tbsp	Tahini (I prefer hulled tahini for taste)
⅓ cup	Boiling water
½	Lemon, juiced

- Mix the ingredients together with a whisk.
- For a thinner consistency, add more water.

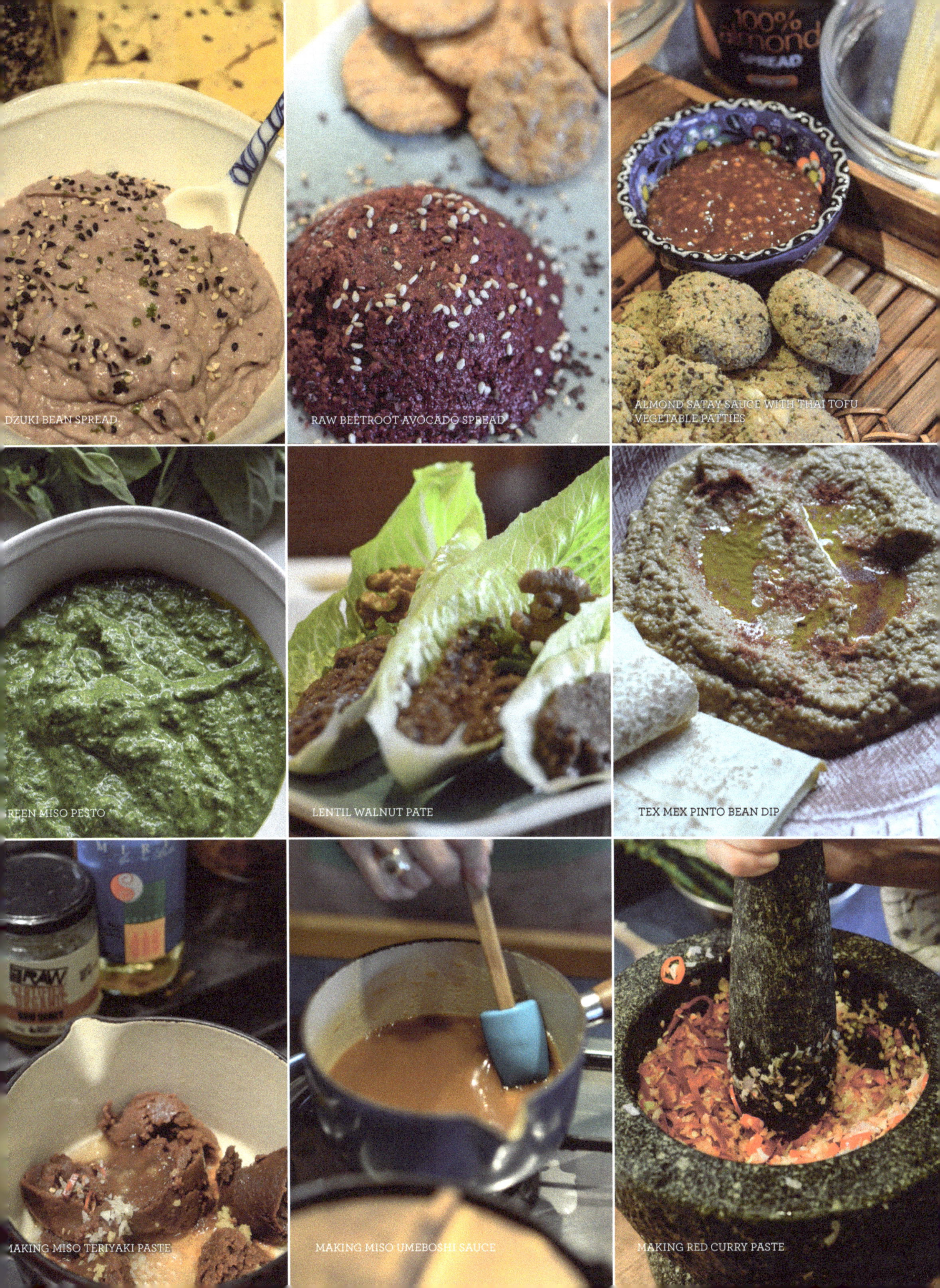

MISO UMEBOSHI SAUCE

A tangy dressing or sauce for noodles,
steamed vegetables, savoury pancakes and patties

MAKES ABOUT 1 CUP
KEEPS REFRIGERATED IN A GLASS JAR FOR 1 WEEK

2 tbsp	Toasted sesame oil
2 tbsp	Tamari
¼ cup	Honey (or any other sweetener, e.g. coconut syrup)
2 tbsp	Brown rice vinegar
1 ½ tbsp	Kuzu starch (dissolved in ¼ cup water)
1 tbsp	Umeboshi plum paste OR 2 tbsp Plum vinegar (I use Spiral Foods Plum Vinegar – Ume Su)
2 tbsp	White miso paste (Shiro)
¼ cup	Warm water heated via kettle or saucepan (don't use warm tap water)

- Combine oil, tamari, honey and brown rice vinegar in a small saucepan.
- Bring slowly to the boil, then add dissolved kuzu starch. Stir in well, and allow the mixture to simmer for 5 minutes, until thick and bubbly. Remove from heat and let it sit to thicken.
- Combine the umeboshi paste or plum vinegar with the miso paste and warm water (to thin). Then stir into the thickened mixture and mix until smooth.
- Serve as a dressing or sauce.

GREEN MISO PESTO

Topping for pasta, noodles and stir-fries

MAKES ABOUT 1 CUP
KEEPS REFRIGERATED IN A GLASS JAR FOR 1 WEEK

150 g	Spinach leaves
1 ½ cups	Fresh basil leaves
50 g	Roasted walnuts, cashews or seeds (yes, you can use pine nuts)
2 small	Garlic cloves, chopped
2 tbsp	Lemon juice
2 tbsp	Miso paste (I like using white Shiro miso here, but for a stronger, saltier flavour you can use darker Genmai or Mugi miso)
2 tbsp	Extra virgin olive oil
As required	Water

- Wash greens and drain.
- Roast nuts in a low, pre-heated oven for 8 to 10 minutes. Remove and allow to cool.
- Place half the spinach and all basil leaves in a food processor and add the remaining ingredients (except for the olive oil). Blend until the mixture is evenly chopped.
- Add the remaining spinach and oil and pulse on and off for a coarse puree consistency. Add a little water if required.
- Serve as desired.

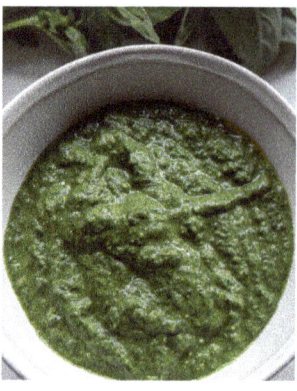

TOFU BEETROOT DIP

MAKES ABOUT 2 CUPS
KEEP REFRIGERATED. BEST USED WITHIN 3 DAYS

250 g	Tofu (soft or firm – it's your choice)
2 large	Beetroot
2–3 tbsp	Tahini, to taste (my students prefer hulled tahini)
2–3 tbsp	Miso paste, to taste (I prefer white Shiro)
2 tbsp	Plum vinegar (I use Spiral Foods Plum vinegar – Ume Su)
2 small	Garlic cloves, minced
8 cm	Wakame sea vegetable

- Cook whole beetroot with skin in enough water to cover for 45 minutes. Drain and cool. Remove skin with hands (wear gloves if you don't want to stain your hands) as the skin will peel off easily.
- Soak wakame in enough water to cover until soft (approx. 10 minutes), remove stem and chop. Keep strained wakame soaking water to add later.
- Soak tofu in boiling water for 5 minutes. Drain.
- Place all ingredients in a food processor and blend until it reaches your desired consistency.
- Add boiling water and strained wakame soaking water as required to make creamier.
- Serve with crackers or vegetable crudités, or on top of steamed vegetables and salads.

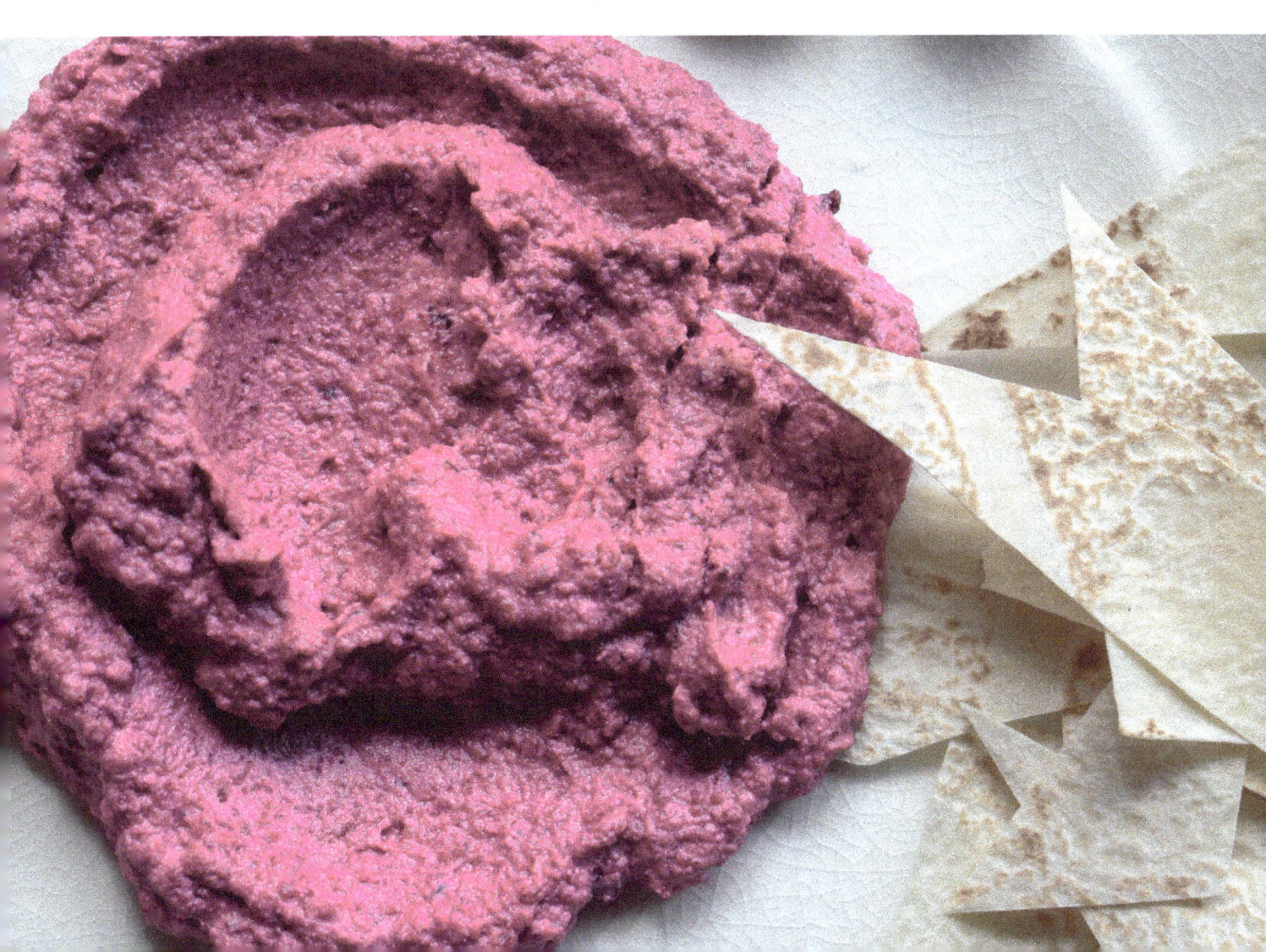

CHICKPEA CELERY HUMMUS
A healthy protein and calcium-rich hummus

MAKES ABOUT 2 CUPS
KEEP REFRIGERATED. BEST USED WITHIN 3 DAYS

2 small	Garlic cloves, minced
2 stalks	Celery, coarsely chopped
⅓ cup	Lemon juice
400 g	Chickpeas, cooked or tinned
¼ cup	Tahini (I like hulled tahini)
1 tsp	Cumin, ground
2 tsp	Tamari or shoyu OR 1 tbsp miso paste (for sweeter taste use white miso; for saltier taste use a darker miso)
Garnish	Extra virgin olive oil
Garnish	Paprika and/or cayenne pepper

- In a food processor, puree the garlic, celery and lemon juice.
- Drain cooked chickpeas or tinned ones. Save cooking liquid or liquid from tin.
- Add the chickpeas, tahini, cumin and tamari, shoyu or miso paste to food processor.
- Process until smooth and creamy. Add saved cooking liquid if required.
- Garnish with a drizzle of extra virgin olive oil and a sprinkle of paprika or cayenne.

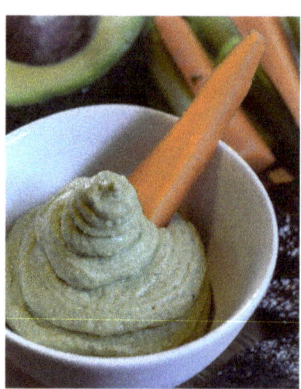

See p.97 for tips on how to cook organic dried beans.

TEX-MEX PINTO BEAN DIP

MAKES ABOUT 2 CUPS
KEEP REFRIGERATED. BEST USED WITHIN 3 DAYS

400 g	Pinto beans, cooked or tinned
2 small	Garlic cloves, minced
2 tbsp	Red onion, minced
1 tbsp	Fresh parsley, finely chopped
½–1 tsp	Ground cumin, to taste
¼ cup	Tomatoes, cooked and diced (or use tomatoes in a BPA-free tin)
1 large	Green jalapeño chilli, seeds removed, chopped
2 tsp	Plum vinegar (I use Spiral Foods Plum Vinegar – Ume Su)

- Place all ingredients in a blender or food processor, and puree until smooth and creamy.
- Serve with crackers, chips, corn tortillas or tacos (see recipe).

Note: If using tinned tomatoes, store the remainder in glass jar in the refrigerator.

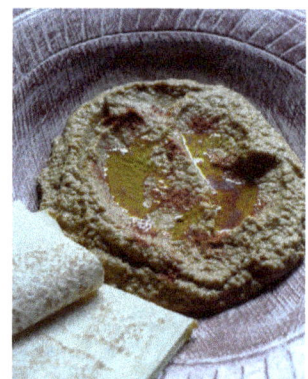

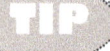

TOASTING SESAME SEEDS

It tastes fresher and better to make your own toasted sesame seeds.

- I make a jar every couple of weeks. Sprinkle on any meals, on rice, in salads, on vegetables.
- In a clean dry saucepan, place 1 cup raw sesame seeds and, on medium heat, stir well with a wooden spoon for a few minutes. Be careful they don't burn.
- Cool then store in a sealed glass jar.

RAW BEETROOT AVOCADO SPREAD

MAKES ABOUT 2 CUPS
KEEP REFRIGERATED. BEST USED WITHIN 3 DAYS

300 g	Beetroots
2	Spring onions, chopped
½	Avocado
½ cup	Fresh coriander, chopped
1 small	Red chilli, dried
3 tbsp	Walnuts
2 tbsp	Extra virgin olive oil
1 tbsp	Apple cider vinegar or lemon juice
To taste	Sea salt and black pepper
Garnish	Dulse flakes (I use Eden Foods)
Garnish	Toasted sesame seeds
Garnish	Fresh mint leaves, chopped

- Scrub beetroot well and trim ends. Chop.
- Place in food processor with all other ingredients (except garnishes).
- Adjust seasonings as required.
- Place in serving bowl. Sprinkle on dulse flakes, toasted sesame seeds and chopped mint leaves.
- Drizzle with olive oil and serve with crackers or veggies, or on top of noodles or vegetable salads.

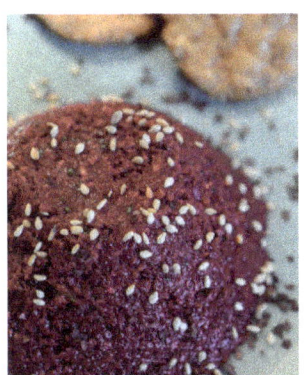

ADZUKI BEAN SPREAD

MAKES ABOUT 2 CUPS
KEEP REFRIGERATED. BEST USED WITHIN 3 DAYS

400 g	Adzuki beans, cooked or tinned
2 tbsp	Tahini
1 tbsp	Umeboshi paste
1–2 tsp	Ginger, grated, to taste
1 tbsp	Miso paste (I like Genmai or Mugi miso)
⅓ cup	Hot water
Garnish	Sea vegetable seasoning (I use Furikake seasoning from Spiral Foods)

- Drain beans and place in blender.
- Dissolve miso in boiled hot water and add to blender with other ingredients.
- Adjust flavour and consistency to taste.
- Spread on wheat-free baked sesame or quinoa rice crackers or savoury pancakes, or enjoy on top of delicious sea vegetable brown rice.

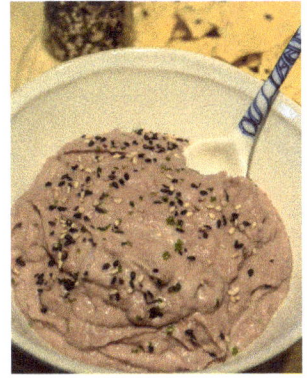

Adzuki beans (also known as aduki or azuki beans) are small, red, dry beans often used in Japanese and Chinese dishes. They're my favourite bean and are regarded as the king of beans in Japan. I have made this recipe for many classes over the years so I know that everyone enjoyed the tasty adzuki bean.

MISO DILL DRESSING
For Kidney Bean Salad

MAKES ABOUT 3/4 CUP
KEEPS REFRIGERATED IN A GLASS JAR FOR 1 WEEK

1 tbsp	White miso paste (Shiro)
2 tbsp	Lemon juice
2 tbsp	Extra virgin olive oil
1 tbsp	Flaxseed oil (optional)
2 tbsp	Dill, fresh, chopped
1 tsp	Tamari or shoyu (optional)
⅓ cup	Water

- Combine all ingredients in a small bowl, mixing well.
- Add to salad and allow to marinate for 15 minutes before serving.
- Any leftover dressing can be stored in glass jar for up to 1 week. Add more water as required.

LIME VINAIGRETTE

MAKES ABOUT 1 CUP
KEEPS REFRIGERATED IN A GLASS JAR FOR 1 WEEK

¼ cup	Lime juice
¼ cup	Extra virgin olive oil
¼ cup	Brown rice vinegar
1 tbsp	Plum vinegar (I use Spiral Foods Plum Vinegar – Ume Su)
1 small	Garlic clove
Pinch	Sea salt
2 tbsp	Warm water or more as required
1 tbsp	Basil, fresh, chopped
1 tbsp	Dill, fresh, chopped

- Combine all ingredients in blender.

SHIITAKE SESAME VINAIGRETTE

MAKES ABOUT 1 CUP

4	Shiitake mushrooms, dried
½ cup	Boiling water
¼ cup	Apple cider vinegar
6	Olives, pitted
2 tsp	Toasted sesame oil
⅓ cup	Extra virgin olive oil
Pinch	Sea salt
2 tsp	Toasted sesame seeds

- Place dried shiitakes in bowl and cover with ½ cup boiling water. Let soak for about 20 minutes, until softened. Remove and discard stems. Keep soaking water.
- Place softened mushrooms in blender with strained soaking water. Add apple cider vinegar and pitted olives. Blend until well chopped.
- Add toasted sesame oil, olive oil and salt. Blend until just combined.
- Remove from blender into glass jar. Add toasted sesame seeds.
- Use on steamed vegetables, salads, stir fries, cooked brown rice, quinoa, noodles.

I prefer the flavour of dried Japanese shiitake mushrooms – see glossary

RED CURRY PASTE
For Thai Tofu Curry

MAKES 1 FULL CUP
KEEPS REFRIGERATED IN A GLASS JAR FOR 2 WEEKS

6 long	Red chillies, fresh
2 tsp	Coriander seeds
5 cm	Galangal, peeled, finely chopped
1	Lemongrass stalk, finely chopped
4	Garlic cloves
1	Shallot, chopped
1 tsp	Lime juice
1 tsp	Sea salt
2 tbsp	Coconut oil

- Put chillies in mortar and crush with pestle, then add garlic and crush it with chillies and then do the same with all other ingredients, finally mixing in the oil.

OR

- Place all ingredients in food processor and blend to a thick paste.

ALMOND SATAY SAUCE
Serve with Thai Tofu Vegetable Patties

MAKES 1 CUP
KEEPS REFRIGERATED FOR 1 WEEK

3 tbsp	Almond butter (I like Melrose almond butter)
1 tsp	Toasted sesame oil
1 tsp	Chilli paste
⅓ cup	Tamari or shoyu
2 tbsp	Coconut syrup, honey or rice syrup
2 tbsp	Lime juice
As required	Water

- Combine almond butter, sesame oil and chilli paste in a bowl (or food processor) and whisk together until blended.
- Then whisk in tamari or shoyu, sweetener and lime juice.
- Add water for a thinner consistency.

MISO TERIYAKI PASTE
Marinade for tofu, vegetables or noodles

KEEPS REFRIGERATED IN A GLASS JAR
FOR UP TO 2 WEEKS

6 tbsp	Dark miso paste
3 tbsp	Mirin
1 tbsp	Ginger, grated
1 tbsp	Garlic, minced
1 tbsp	Honey
optional	Chilli, crushed, to taste

- Place all ingredients into a heavy-based saucepan and mix slowly over low heat for about 3 minutes.
- Allow to cool before placing in glass jar to store in refrigerator.
- Dilute desired amount of paste with water before using.

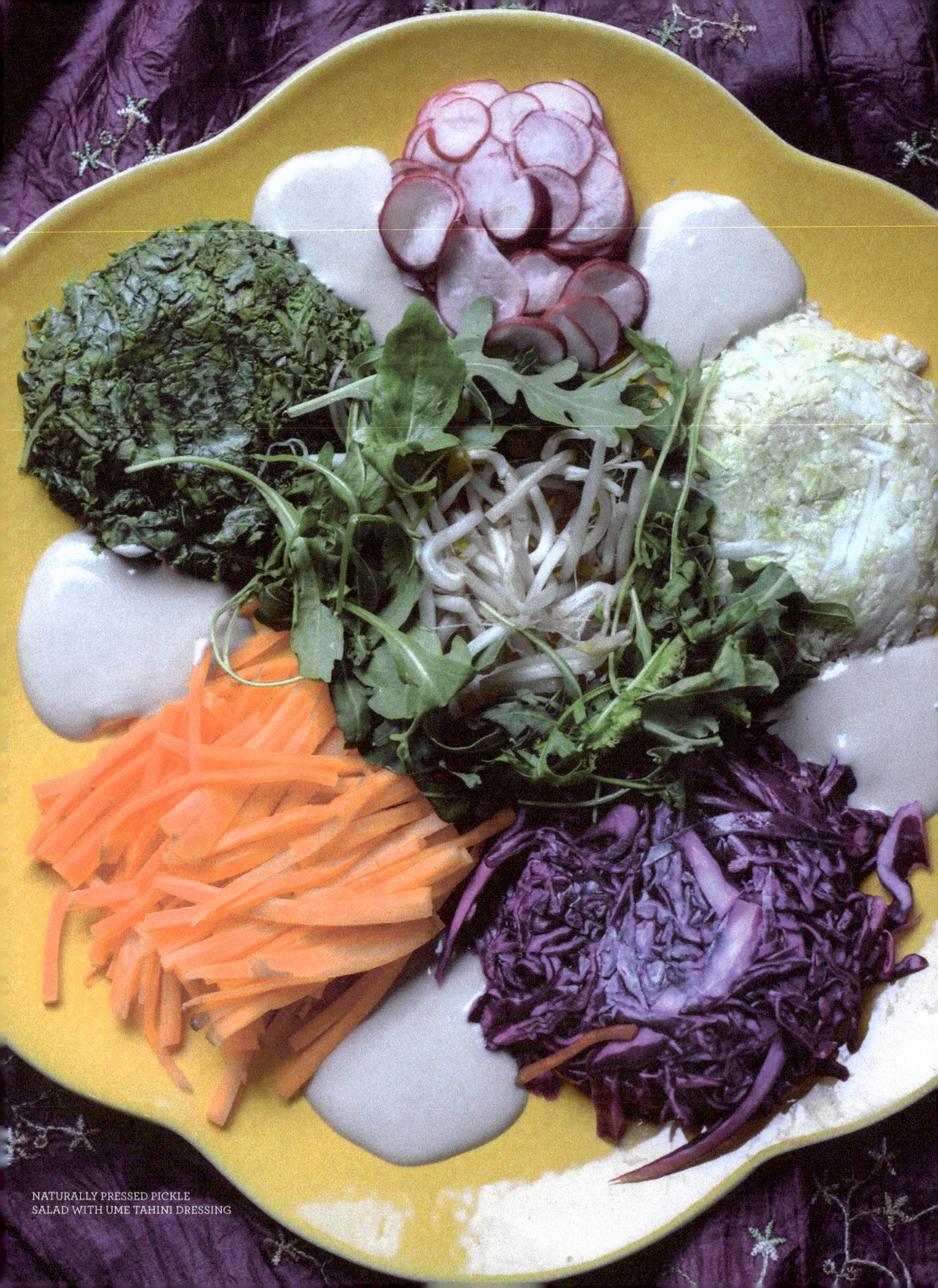

NATURALLY PRESSED PICKLE SALAD WITH UME TAHINI DRESSING

Greens : Salads : Sea Vegetables

Naturally Pressed Pickle Salad 47

Pickled Cabbage 49

Sweet And Sour Quick Pickles 49

Sweet And Sour Arame 51

Spring Salad.. 52

Spinach Roll with Sesame Dressing 55

Simply Boiled Kale with Creamy Ginger Dressing 57

Cucumber Wakame Salad 57

Brown Rice Sushi Rolls – Norimaki 59

Nori Pyramids – Onigiri 61

Coconut Tofu Snake Beans.. 63

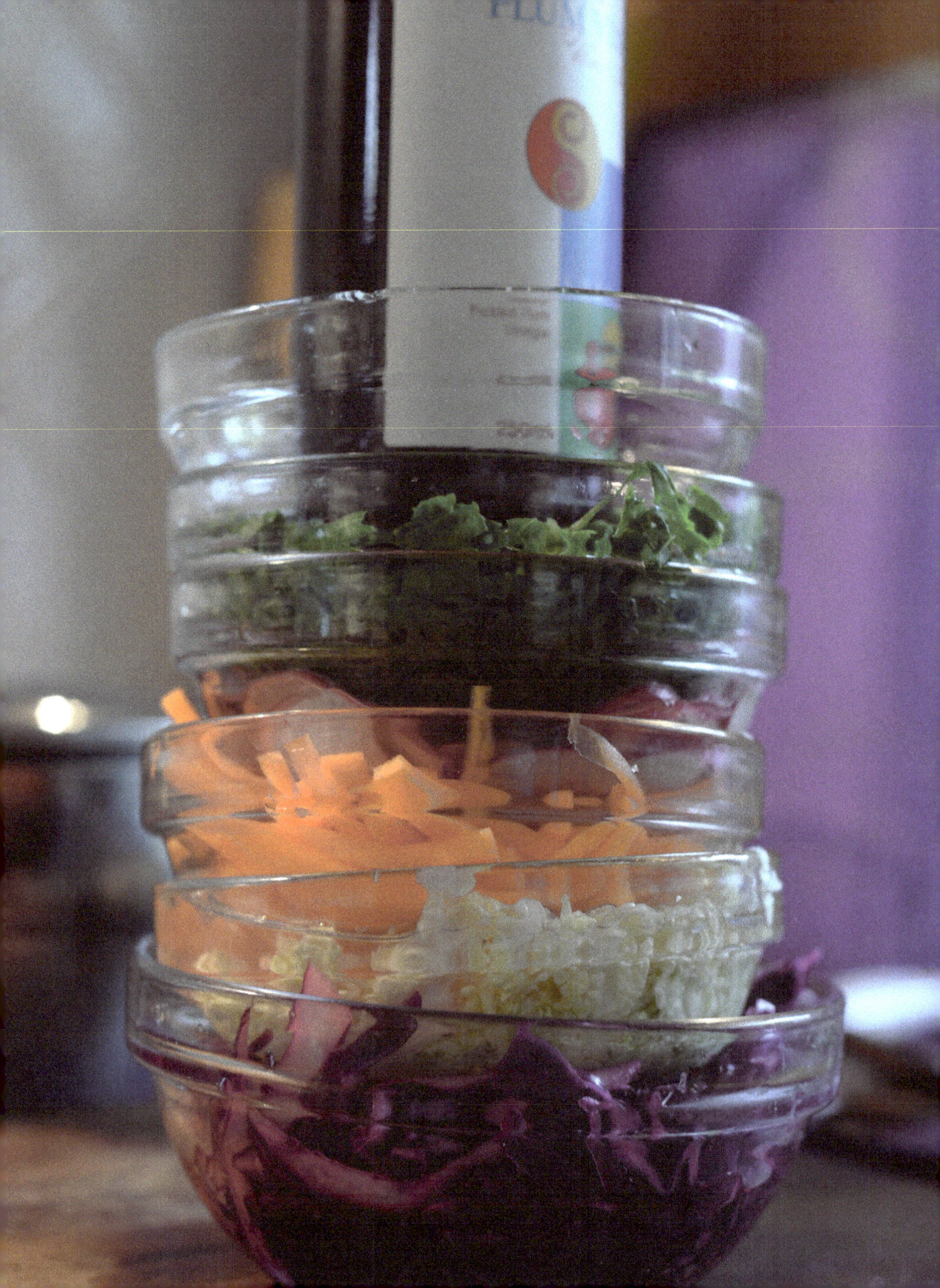

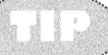 **PRESSED SALADS**

Pressed salad is thinly sliced vegetables lightly pickled with sea salt, shoyu, apple cider vinegar, brown rice vinegar or plum vinegar (Ume Su). Vegetables are pressed with a pickle press or in a crock pressed with a weighted plate or with this method in recipe.

Any raw vegetables can be used in this recipe as they are quite literally 'pressed' or marinated with alkalising plum vinegar and fermented apple cider vinegar until the raw and watery quality is released and removed. This method preserves vegetables and helps break down tough cellulose walls of raw foods, ensuring good absorption of vitamins and minerals.

Naturally made pickles promote salivations and have enzymes that help break down and digest foods, especially wholegrains.

There are a few processes in this recipe. If you don't have a pickle press, using small glass bowls placed on top of each other is a good way to press.

For more information about the Japanese Pickle Press that I use please check out www.mywholefoodcommunity.com and search for Japanese Pickle Press.

NATURALLY PRESSED PICKLE SALAD
With Ume Tahini Dressing

MAKES A LARGE PLATTER
KEEPS PICKLING IN REFRIGERATOR FOR 1 WEEK

½ cup	Red cabbage, thinly sliced
¼ cup	Carrot, julienned
¼ cup	Radish, sliced into rounds
3 tsp	Plum vinegar (I use Spiral Foods Plum Vinegar – Ume Su)
¼ cup	Chinese cabbage, thinly sliced
¼ cup	Kale, thinly sliced
1 cup	Bean shoots
1½ tbsp	Apple cider vinegar
As required	Sea salt
½ cup	Rocket leaves

UME TAHINI DRESSING

4 tbsp	Tahini (I prefer hulled tahini)
¼ cup	Plum vinegar (I use Spiral Foods Plum Vinegar – Ume Su)
⅓ cup	Water

- Place red cabbage in a bowl or pickle press with 1 tsp of the plum vinegar and 1 tsp of sea salt. Mix well. Then cover with another small bowl or plate.
- Place carrots in another bowl and repeat the same process.
- Place radish in another bowl and repeat the process again.
- Place Chinese cabbage in a bowl with ½ tbsp of the apple cider vinegar and 1 tsp of salt. Mix well. Then cover with another small bowl or plate.
- Place kale in another bowl and repeat the same process as with cabbage.
- Place bean shoots in another bowl and repeat the process again as with cabbage.
- Leave all vegetables to press (marinate) for 30 minutes or more, until the liquid begins to release.
- While above vegetables are pressing, wash and drain the rocket.
- Drain all bowls of excess liquid.
- Place drained pressed ingredients on a large serving platter.
- Garnish with the rocket leaves.
- Make ume tahini dressing to drizzle on salad.

DRESSING

- Place tahini, plum vinegar and water into a mixing bowl and stir mixture until it becomes creamy.
- Add additional water to make a thinner dressing.
- Adjust plum vinegar amount to taste.

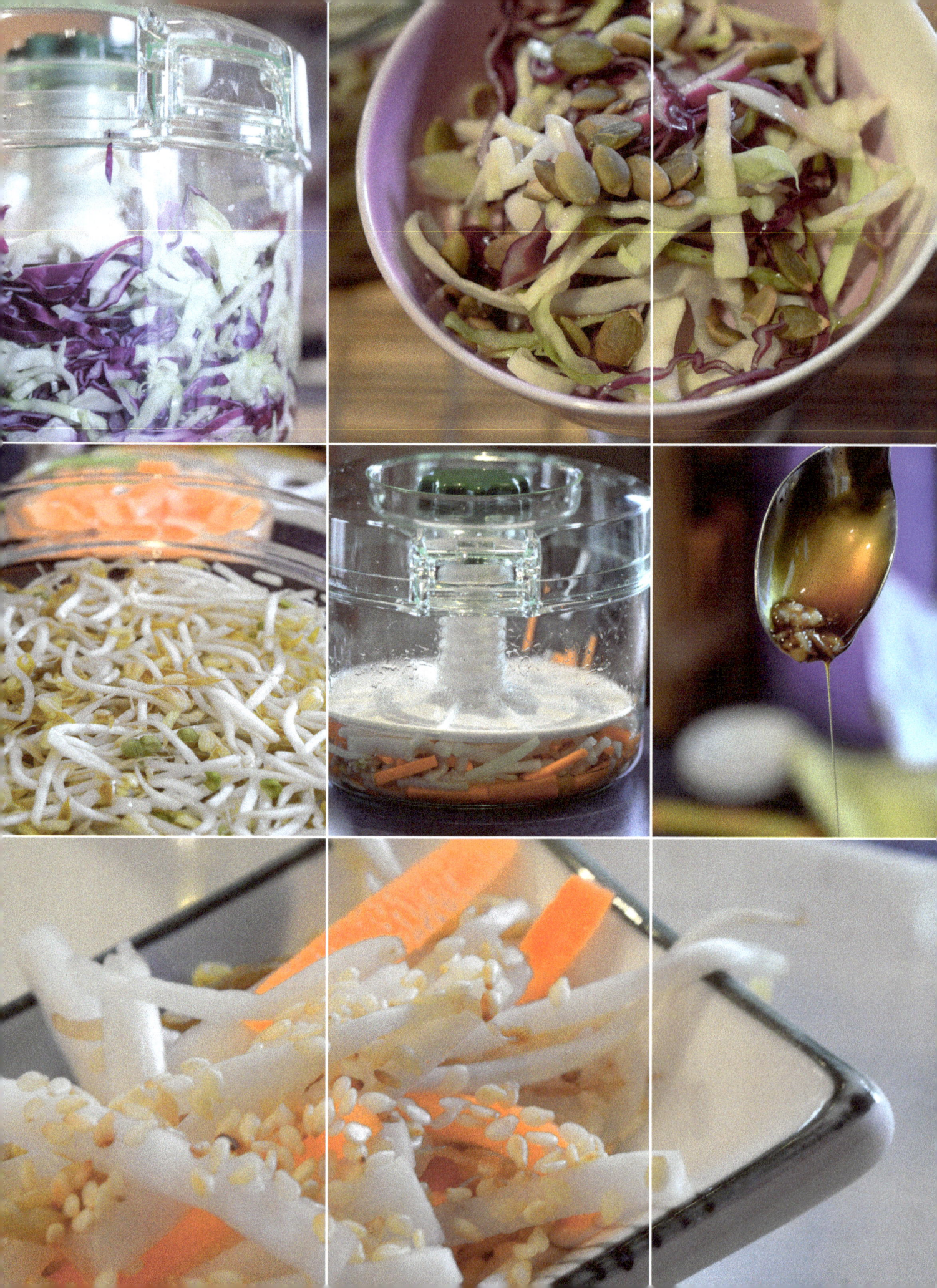

PICKLED CABBAGE

MAKES ABOUT 4 CUPS
KEEPS REFRIGERATED FOR 1 WEEK

¼ small	Red cabbage
½ small	Green cabbage
2	Spring onions, finely chopped (optional)
2 tbsp	Plum vinegar (I use Spiral Foods Plum Vinegar – Ume Su) or lemon juice
2 tsp	Sea salt
Garnish	Parsley, finely chopped
Garnish	Roasted pumpkin or sunflower seeds

- Slice both cabbages into 2 cm slices. Wash then pat dry.
- Mix well with your hands the cabbage, spring onions (if using), plum vinegar or lemon juice and sea salt.
- Press cabbage using a plate with a weight on top or use a pickle press.
- Let sit covered with a cloth at room temperature for a day. Make sure that the water released from the cabbage covers the mix. If not, add ½ cup more water.
- Serve with garnishes.

TIP: These pickles are more delicious if aged at room temperature for 2–3 days. Pickles can then be refrigerated.

SWEET AND SOUR QUICK PICKLES

SERVES 2–3
KEEPS REFRIGERATED FOR UP TO 1 WEEK

1 tsp	Sea salt
4 tbsp	Brown rice vinegar, apple cider vinegar or plum vinegar
2 tbsp	Rice syrup, coconut syrup or honey
1 medium	Carrot
1 small	Daikon radish
1 cup	Bean shoots, washed and drained
3 tbsp	Toasted sesame seeds

- Mix sea salt, vinegar and sweetener in a bowl.
- Finely grate carrot and daikon or cut into fine matchsticks and add, with bean shoots, to vinegar mix.
- Allow mixture to marinate for at least 30 minutes before serving. (You can use a pickle press or place in glass bowl with a smaller glass bowl pressed on top to keep the vegetables submerged.)
- Sprinkle with toasted sesame seeds (see tip on p.40).

For more information about the Japanese Pickle Press that I use please check out www.mywholefoodcommunity.com and search for Japanese Pickle Press.

This recipe was shared at the very first traditional Japanese cooking class at my Japanese Cooking School in 1986. I took the recipe given to me by Japanese Master Chef Itosan (Osamu Ito) and adjusted it for macrobiotic and healthy food enthusiasts using Spiral Foods ingredients.

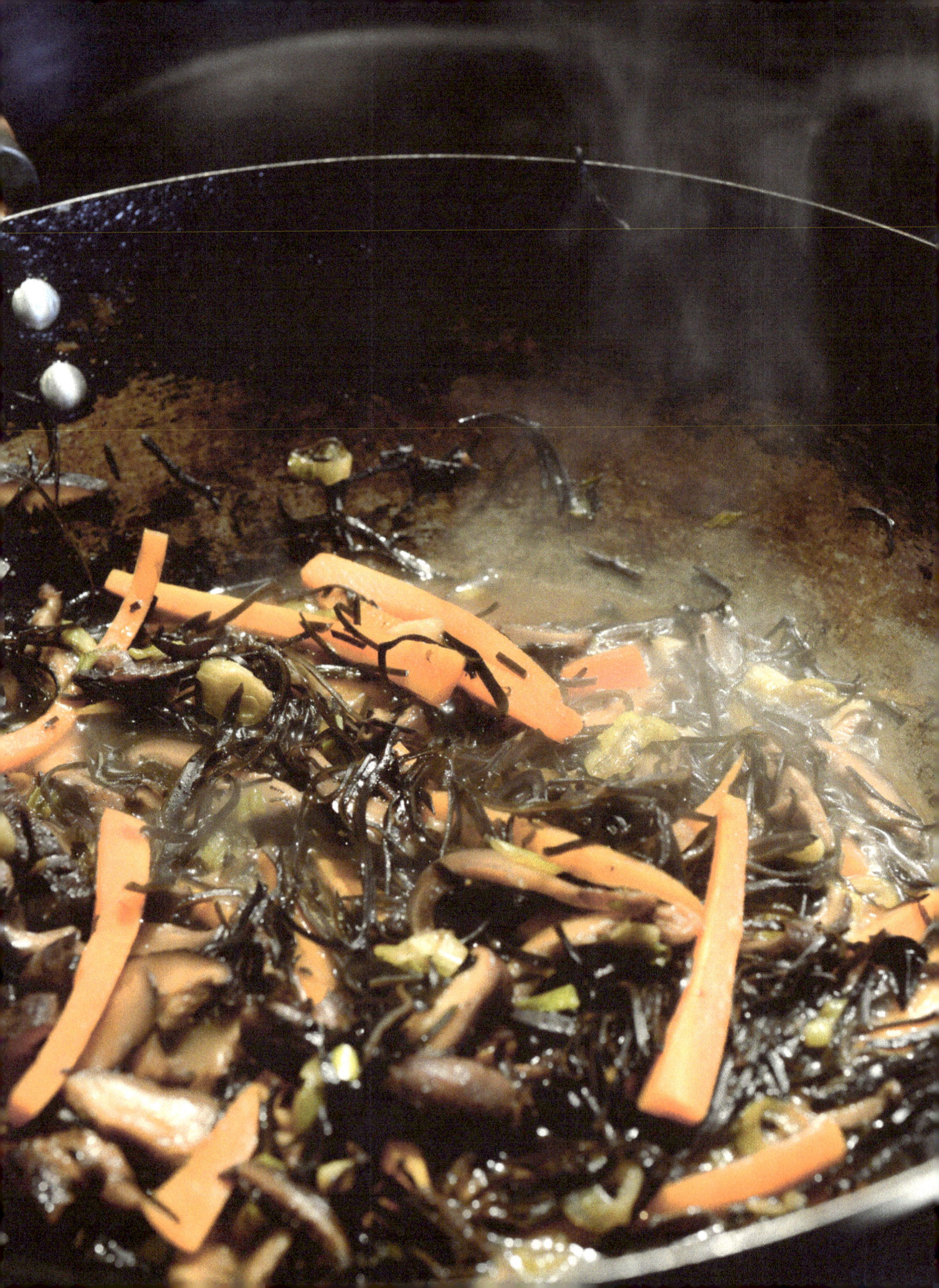

SWEET AND SOUR ARAME

MAKES 4-6 SERVINGS
KEEPS REFRIGERATED FOR 1 WEEK

½ cup	Arame sea vegetable
1 cup	Shiitake mushrooms, dried
1 tbsp	Sesame oil
3 tbsp	Coconut syrup or honey
½ cup	Carrots, julienned
1	Spring onion, finely chopped
2 tbsp	Apple cider vinegar
1 tbsp	Tamari or shoyu
2 tbsp	Toasted sesame seeds

For this recipe the flavour of dried Japanese shiitake mushrooms is preferred – see picture in glossary.

- In a medium bowl, soak arame in 1 cup water to cover for 10 minutes. Strain.
- Soak mushrooms in 2 cups boiled hot water for at least 20 minutes. Drain mushrooms, reserve soaking water. Cut off stems and discard; slice mushroom caps.
- Warm sesame oil in a heavy-based wok or frypan over moderate heat. Add softened arame and cook for 5 minutes, stirring occasionally. Add sweetener, matchstick carrots, finely chopped spring onion, vinegar, tamari or shoyu and chopped mushrooms. Pour in enough strained mushroom soaking water to cover ingredients (add a little more water if not enough to cover).
- Raise the heat and bring mixture to boil then lower heat and simmer uncovered until nearly all cooking liquid has evaporated and arame is tender.
- Serve hot or cold over greens, with chickpea polenta, wholegrains or in sandwiches.

This is a nutritionally highly concentrated and rich flavoured side dish so best serve only 2–3 tbsp per person.

SPRING SALAD
With Plum Basil Dressing

SERVES 3-4

SALAD

8 cm	Wakame sea vegetable
3 stalks	Celery, 5 cm julienne
4	Red radishes, sliced into rounds
3	Spring onions, finely chopped
2 tbsp	Tamari or shoyu
4 leaves	Cos lettuce, sliced
1 cup	Watercress or rocket (arugula), chopped
½ cup	Walnuts, roasted and crushed

PLUM BASIL DRESSING

1 tsp	Umeboshi paste OR 1 tbsp Plum vinegar (I use Spiral Foods Plum Vinegar – Ume Su)
3 tbsp	Flaxseed oil (use extra virgin olive oil if you don't have flaxseed oil)
½ cup	Water
6	Basil leaves, fresh, finely chopped

- Soak wakame in enough water to cover until soft (approx. 10 minutes), remove stem and chop. Set aside to drain.
- Place chopped celery, radishes and spring onions in salad bowl and sprinkle with tamari or shoyu. Marinate for 15 minutes or more.
- To make the dressing: In a small bowl mix oil into umeboshi paste or vinegar, then mix in water. Add finely chopped basil.
- Add the lettuce, watercress or rocket, wakame, walnuts and dressing to marinated celery, radishes and spring onions, and serve.

TIP: You can keep this salad in the refrigerator for a couple of days and keep the dressing in a jar to use before serving.

A weekly favourite for me are Sandra's broccoli pancakes. Not only are they easy to make but are light and alkalising and make a perfect meal after some exercise. I thoroughly enjoy participating in one of Sandra's cooking courses once or twice a year – she researches food and encourages us to enjoy meals that feed the body with the phytonutrients, minerals, vitamins and antioxidants. With Sandra being a natural health food advocate, having 30 years of industry expertise and constantly updating her skills with overseas culinary institute training, we can rely on her whole-heartedly to keep us well and disease-free for years!

Melinda Lewis, Melbourne

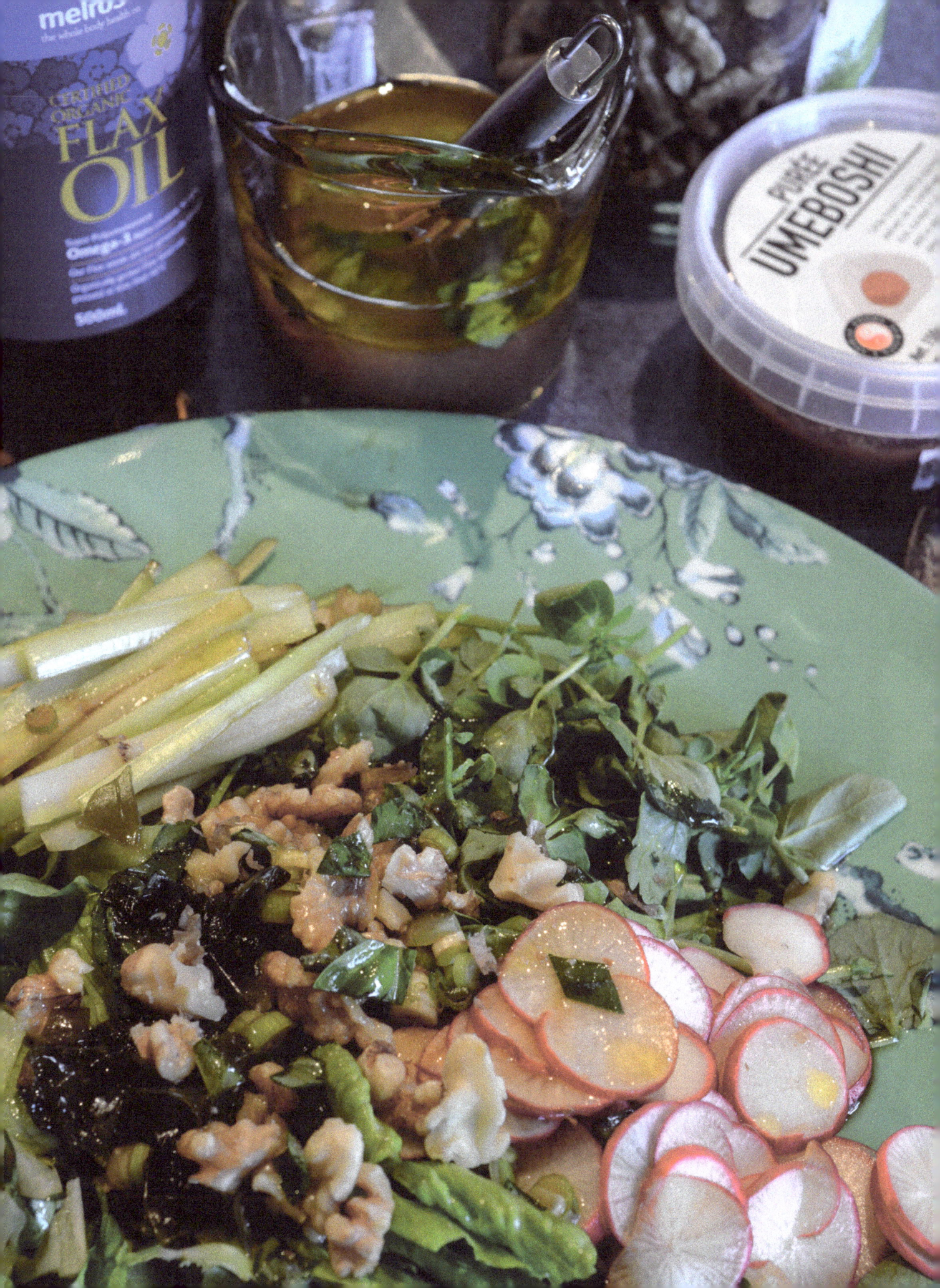

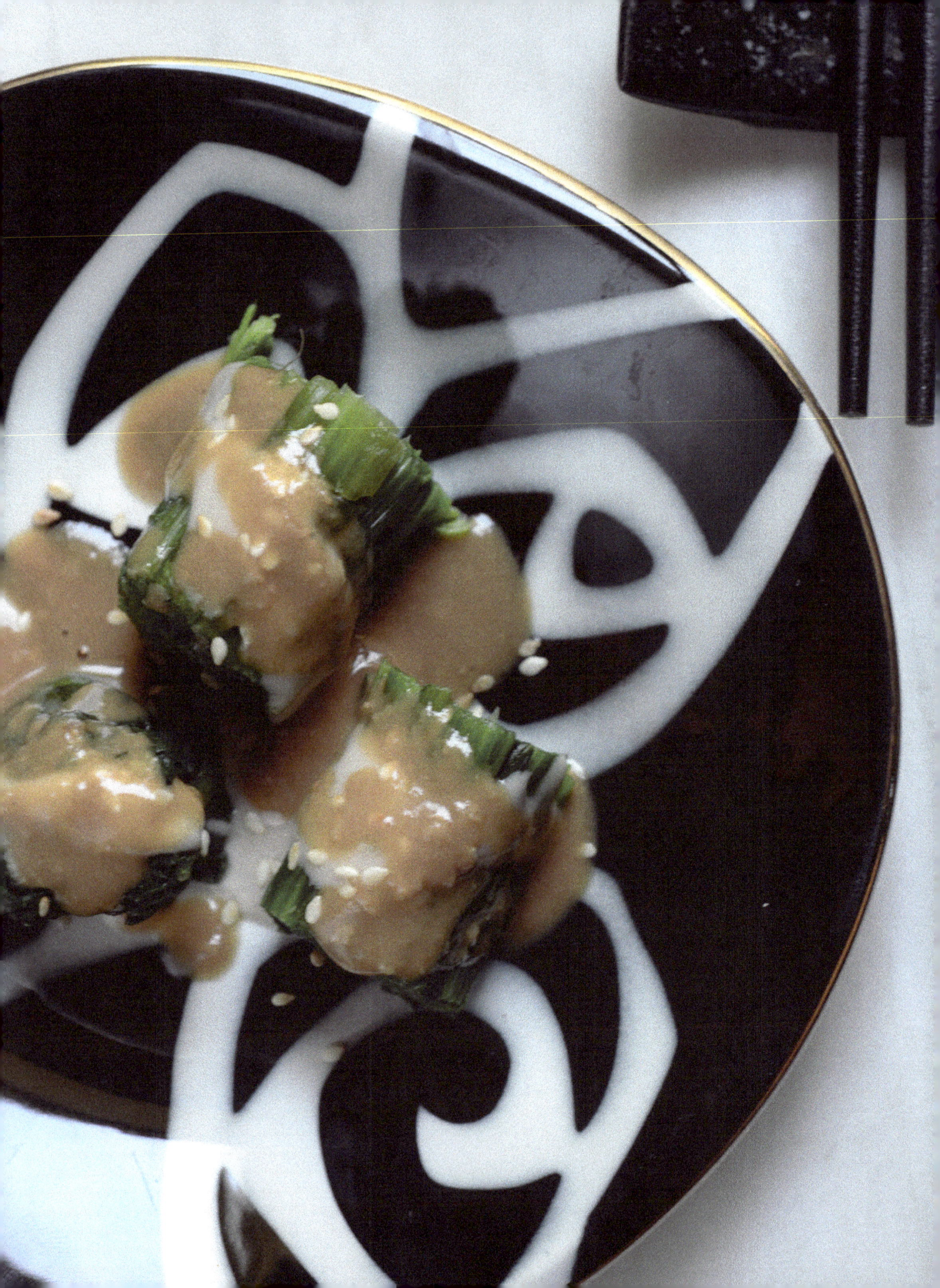

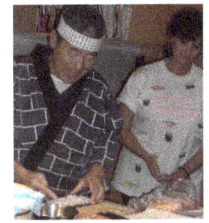

Japanese Master Chef Itosan (Osamu Ito) taught me this recipe in 1986 when we started the Japanese Cooking School in Melbourne. This green side dish is a class favourite.

SPINACH ROLL WITH SESAME DRESSING
Horenso No Goma-Ae

MAKES 8-10 PIECES

1 bunch	Fresh spinach with roots
Pinch	Sea salt

SESAME DRESSING

3 tbsp	Sesame seeds, toasted
2 tbsp	Tahini (I prefer hulled tahini)
1 tsp	Rice syrup
2 tsp	Tamari or shoyu
4–5 tbsp	Water (or use shiitake stock – see below)

MAKING SHIITAKE STOCK

Soak 4 dried shiitake in 2 cups boiled water until softened (the longer the better). Strain to remove grit. This is shiitake stock. You can freeze this in ice cube trays for further use. Use shiitake mushrooms in other recipes.

- Wash spinach thoroughly to remove all traces of grit, leaving all stems and roots intact and still bunched together.
- Bring a large saucepan of water to boil and add pinch of sea salt.
- Add the bunch of spinach, roots first, and boil for 1 minute until roots are tender and leaves have softened. Remove from water and then rinse immediately with cold water. Drain.
- Place enough spinach for roll (about 4 cm diameter), roots at one end, onto sushi mat and roll up, squeezing the spinach in the mat to drain the water. Keep the spinach in the mat for at least 10 minutes to drain fully. Slice off roots.
- To make the dressing: Grind toasted sesame seeds to paste, then add tahini. Add syrup and tamari or shoyu and enough water to make a sauce
- Remove spinach from mat, slice into about 5 cm pieces.
- Serve spinach rolls with dressing.

TIP: You can make this in advance and store whole roll, before slicing, in an airtight container in the refrigerator for 2 days before serving.

This classic Japanese spinach roll combines nutty sesame seeds with spinach for added flavour.

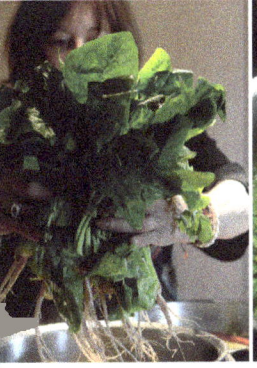 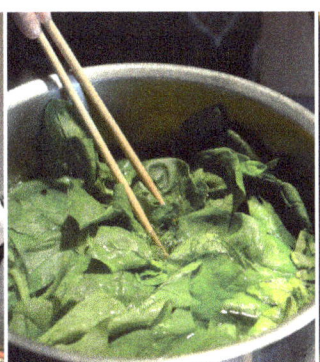 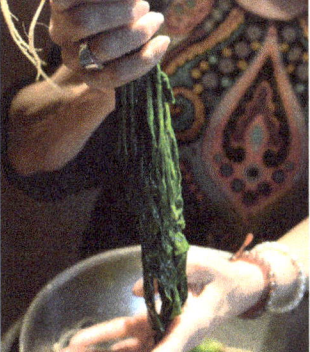 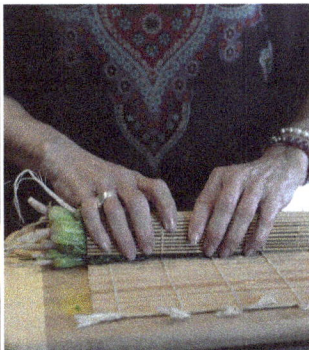 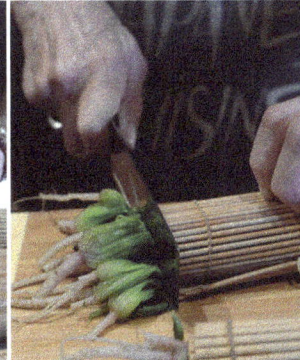

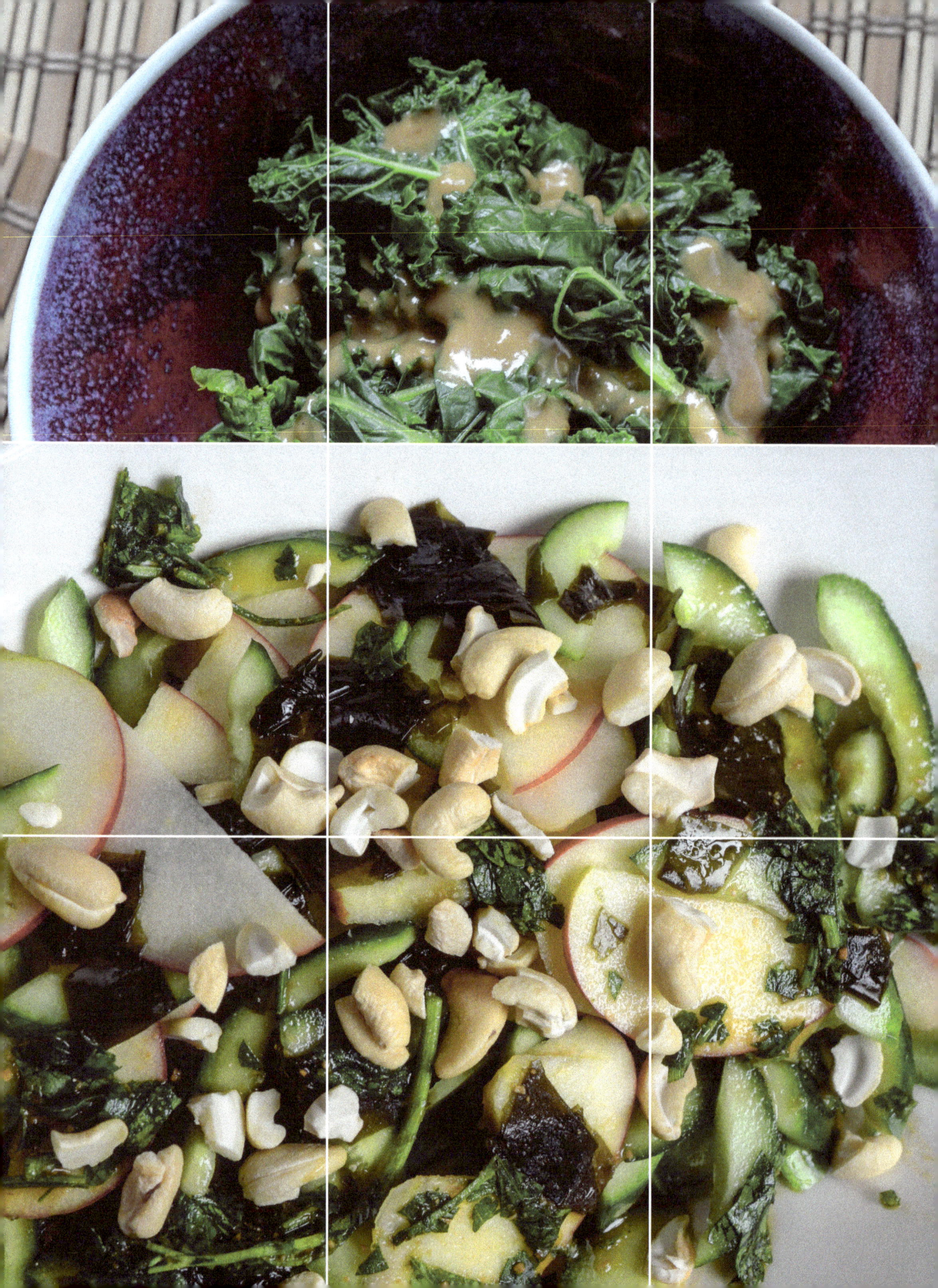

SIMPLY BOILED KALE
With Creamy Ginger Dressing

SERVES 3–4

KALE

1 bunch	Kale
5 cm	Wakame sea vegetable

CREAMY GINGER DRESSING
MAKES 2 CUPS
KEEPS REFRIGERATED FOR UP TO 1 WEEK

4 cloves	Garlic, crushed
¼ cup	Ginger, grated
¼ cup	Tamari
¼ cup	Hulled tahini
¼ cup	Water
2 tbsp	White miso paste (Shiro)
2 tbsp	Rice syrup or other liquid sweetener
2	Spring onions, sliced thinly

- Remove tough stems from kale. Place in large saucepan of boiling water with wakame strip.
- Do not cover saucepan. Return to boil and cook until remaining stems bend easily.
- Drain kale and chop into bite-sized pieces. You can also eat the wakame – simply chop with the kale.
- Dress, then serve.

DRESSING
- Blend all ingredients in a food processor.
- Add more water for thinner consistency.

Use endive, chicory, Chinese broccoli or bok choy in place of kale.

CUCUMBER WAKAME SALAD

SERVES 3–4
KEEPS REFRIGERATED FOR 3 DAYS

SALAD

5 cm	Wakame sea vegetable or Muso/Spiral Foods sea vegetable salad mix
2 medium	Lebanese cucumbers, seeded and thinly sliced
1 small	Red apple, seeded and thinly sliced

MARINADE
MAKES 1 CUP
KEEPS REFRIGERATED IN A GLASS JAR FOR UP TO 1 WEEK

1 tbsp	Miso paste (I like Genmai miso)
1 tbsp	Mirin
2 tsp	Brown rice vinegar
3 tbsp	Parsley, fresh, chopped
⅓ cup	Water
3 tbsp	Orange juice, freshly squeezed
Garnish	Roasted cashews, crushed

- Soak wakame in enough water to cover until soft (approx. 10 minutes), remove stem and chop. Place in a bowl with the sliced apples and cucumber.
- To make the marinade: Place all ingredients for the marinade into a blender. Puree until smooth and creamy.
- Pour ⅓ cup (or as required) over the salad ingredients, mix thoroughly and marinate for 1 hour.
- Pour off marinade and place salad in a serving bowl.
- Garnish with roasted cashew pieces.

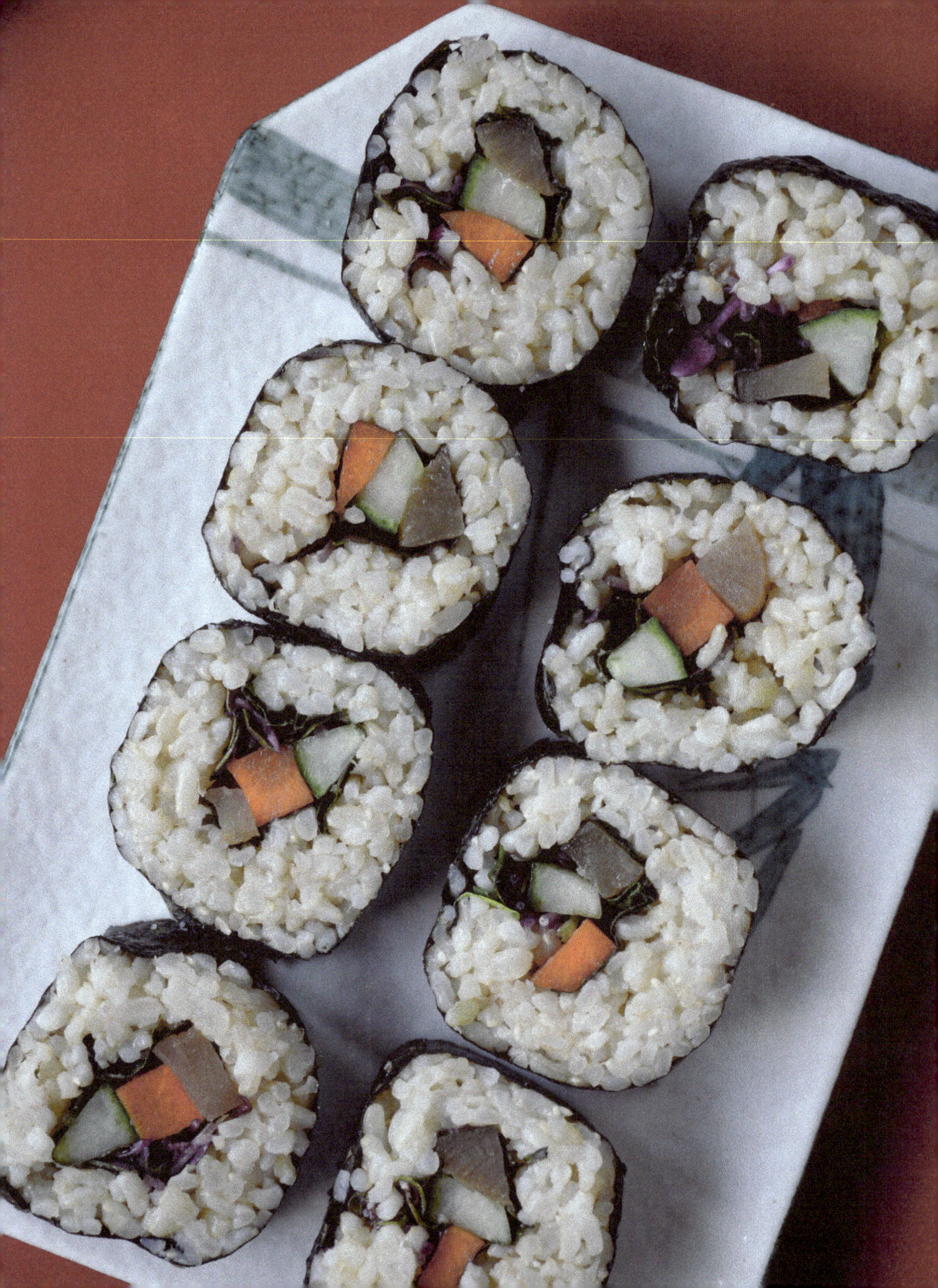

BROWN RICE SUSHI ROLLS – NORIMAKI

SERVES 4

2 cups	Cooked brown rice for sushi (see recipe in Wholegrains section)
6 tbsp	Vinegar mixture (see recipe for cooked brown rice for sushi p.83)
4–6	Sushi nori sheets
1 packet	Pickled daikon radish (I use Spiral Foods takuan, which is daikon radish naturally pickled in rice bran. Wash off rice bran before using)
1	Cucumber, continental or Lebanese, seeded
1	Avocado
1	Carrot or zucchini, cut into strips
To taste	Wasabi (I use Spiral Foods natural wasabi powder diluted with a little water)
Optional	Fresh herbs, shiso leaves or microgreens, to taste
To taste	Pickled ginger
To taste	Tamari or shoyu

PREPARING INGREDIENTS

- Marinate carrot or zucchini strips in a small amount of tamari or shoyu and water for 2 minutes, or until softened. Drain vegetables and place on a platter.
- Slice cucumber, avocado and washed takuan into thin strips and prepare fresh herbs and microgreens. Place on a platter.

ROLLING NORIMAKI

- To roll, place a sheet of sushi nori, rough side up, narrow side horizontal, on a bamboo sushi mat.
- Dampen your hands by dipping them in a bowl of water and shaking off excess (this helps to avoid rice from sticking to your hands), then pack a thin, even layer of rice over the nori. Leave a top edge of about 2 cm without rice. Make sure the rice is not too thick or your roll with be too full of rice without room for fillings.
- Place a variety of fillings (e.g. wasabi first, then cucumber, carrot, avocado, microgreens) in a line about ⅓ of the way up the rice edge closest to you.
- Place thumbs under bamboo mat and fingers on top of fillings and roll the mat over the ingredients, compress ingredients into the roll then lift off bamboo mat and then continue to roll until fully rolled up.
- Compress into a square shape – it will round out once nori gets moist.
- Let roll rest for a few minutes before cutting. Each roll will slice into 6 to 8 pieces. Use a sharp knife.
- Serve immediately with traditional pickled ginger and more wasabi paste as desired. Dip lightly into tamari or shoyu and eat!

EATING TIP: Tamari has a strong, sharp flavour and is ideal for cooking but shoyu is milder and tastier for sushi. Don't dip your sushi too much as it will be too salty and you won't notice the subtle flavour of all the other ingredients.

STORAGE TIP: Once sliced, these rolls are best eaten fresh. If you don't cut the rolls, you can store them by wrapping them up air tight and keeping in the refrigerator until the next day. However, flavour and texture will be compromised.

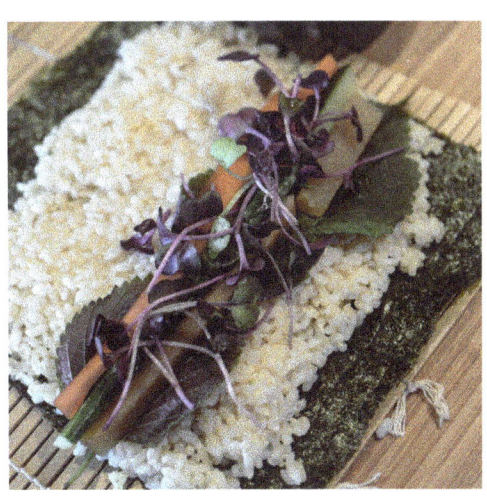

You know that you love cooking equipment, so go out and buy a bamboo sushi mat, hangiri wooden rice bowl with bamboo rice paddle and a hand fan, not only to keep you cool, but to cool down rice.

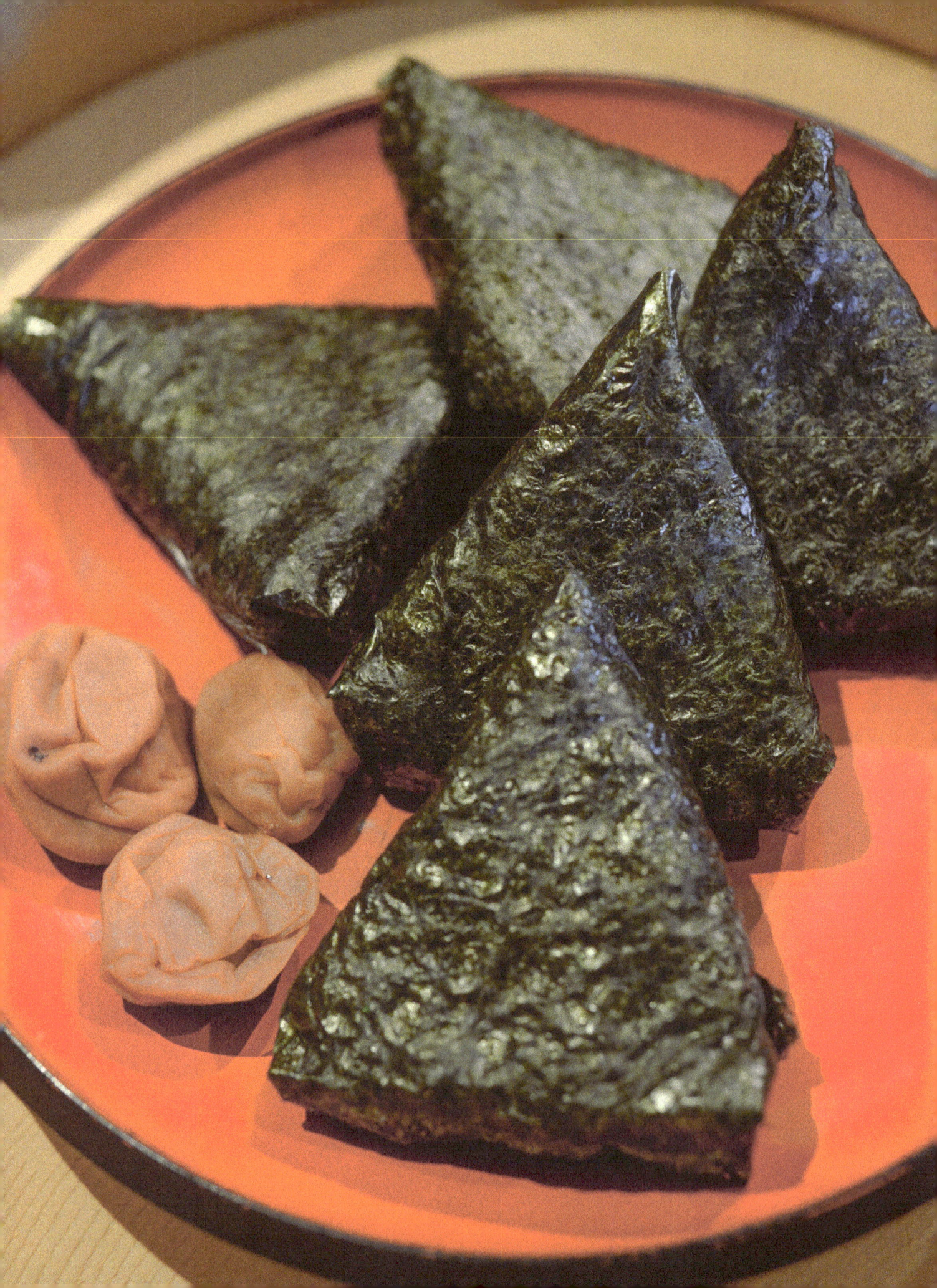

NORI PYRAMIDS – ONIGIRI

MAKES ABOUT 10–12
KEEPS REFRIGERATED IN AIRTIGHT CONTAINER
FOR UP TO 2 DAYS

2 cups	Cooked brown rice for sushi (p.83)
4–6	Sushi nori sheets
1–2 tbsp	Toasted sesame seeds
2–3 tbsp	Umeboshi paste or other fillings, such as a little avocado and cucumber

- Cut nori sheets in half along the longer side.
- Sprinkle toasted sesame seeds into cooked rice.
- Make a triangular shape of rice to fit into the palm of your hand.
- Place this rice triangle in centre of a half nori sheet, add umeboshi paste or other fillings into the centre of the rice triangle and fold as per the photographs.

TIP: Umeboshi has natural antibacterial qualities, so is the ideal filling for onigiri that have to be kept for some time – such as ones made the evening before to eat for lunch the next day.

Tamari has a strong, sharp flavour and is ideal for cooking but shoyu is milder and tastier for sushi. Don't dip sushi too much as it will be too salty and you won't notice the subtle flavour of all the other ingredients.

This was a big favourite in the cafe of my health food store, Manna Natural Foods, almost 30 years ago!

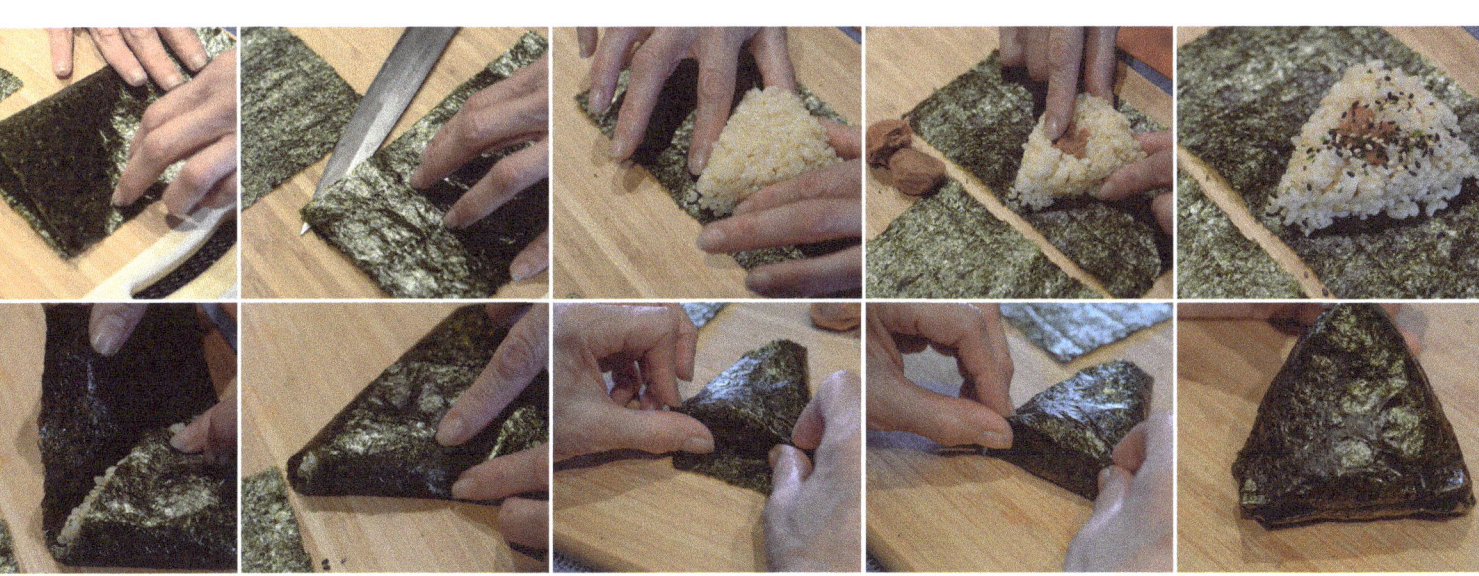

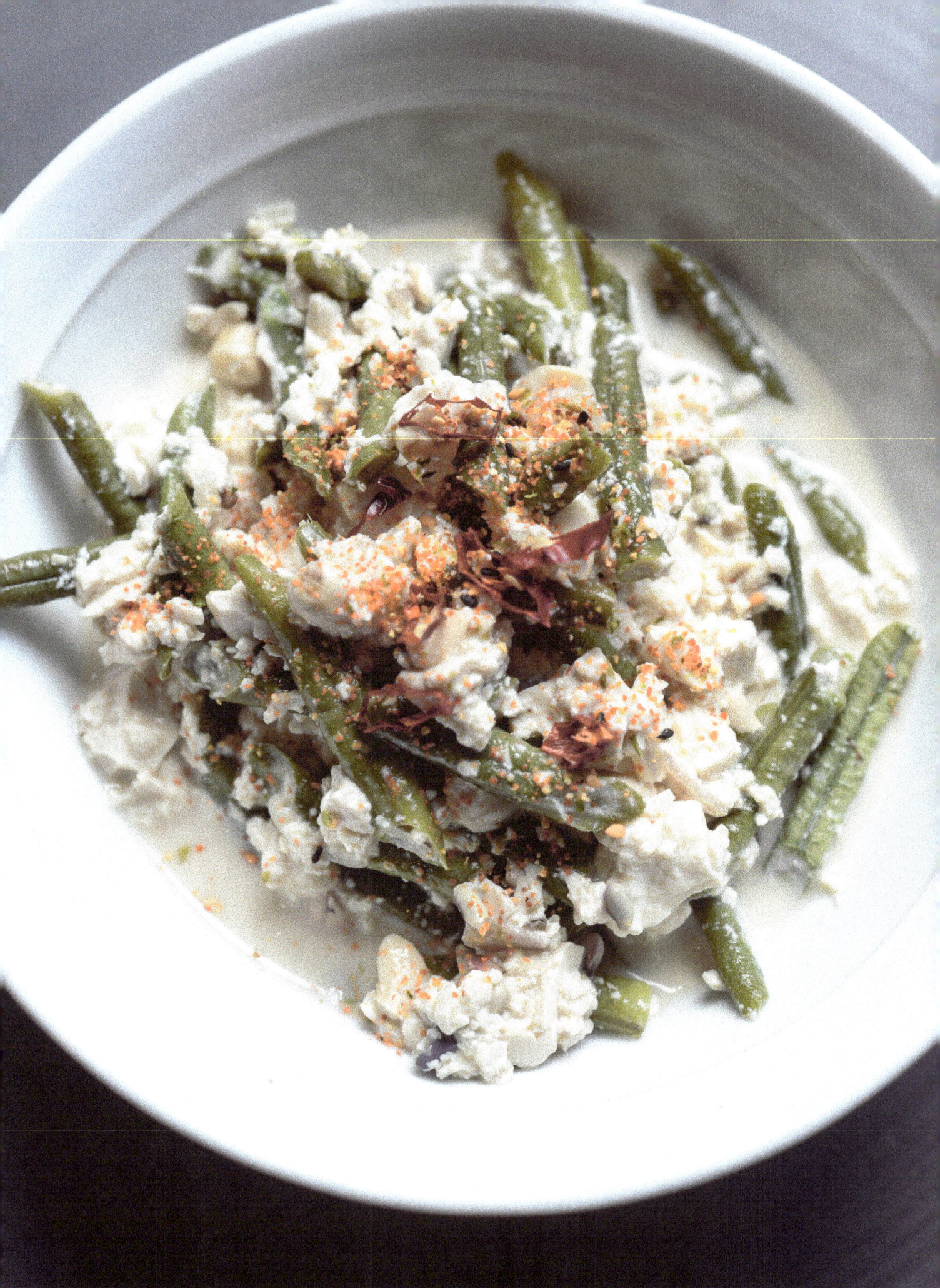

COCONUT TOFU SNAKE BEANS

SERVES 2-3
KEEPS REFRIGERATED FOR UP TO 2 DAYS

200 g	Snake beans or string beans
325 g	Silken tofu
200 ml	Coconut milk
1	Shallot, sliced
25 g	Roasted cashews, crushed
1 tbsp	Lime juice
1 tsp	Coconut sugar
2 tbsp	Tamari or shoyu
1 tsp	Sea salt
Garnish	Chilli flakes, dried

- Slice or cut beans into 3 to 5 cm lengths then simmer in salted water for 2 minutes. Drain.
- Soften the tofu in coconut milk over gentle heat.
- Remove from heat, stir in cooked beans and the rest of ingredients.
- Garnish with chilli flakes.
- This can be served at room temperature.

We are fortunate to have Sandra available to pass on knowledge and information to people wishing to enjoy 'real live food' and assist in healing ourselves with 'food as medicine'. What I always find in Sandra's presentations is her belief in what she teaches, her absolute enthusiasm and an encyclopaedic knowledge of food, its chemical compositions and combination of ingredients to make cooking and eating an exciting and enjoyable experience – you cannot wait to try the food that jumps out at you.

George Viet, Shiatsu Practitioner, Melbourne

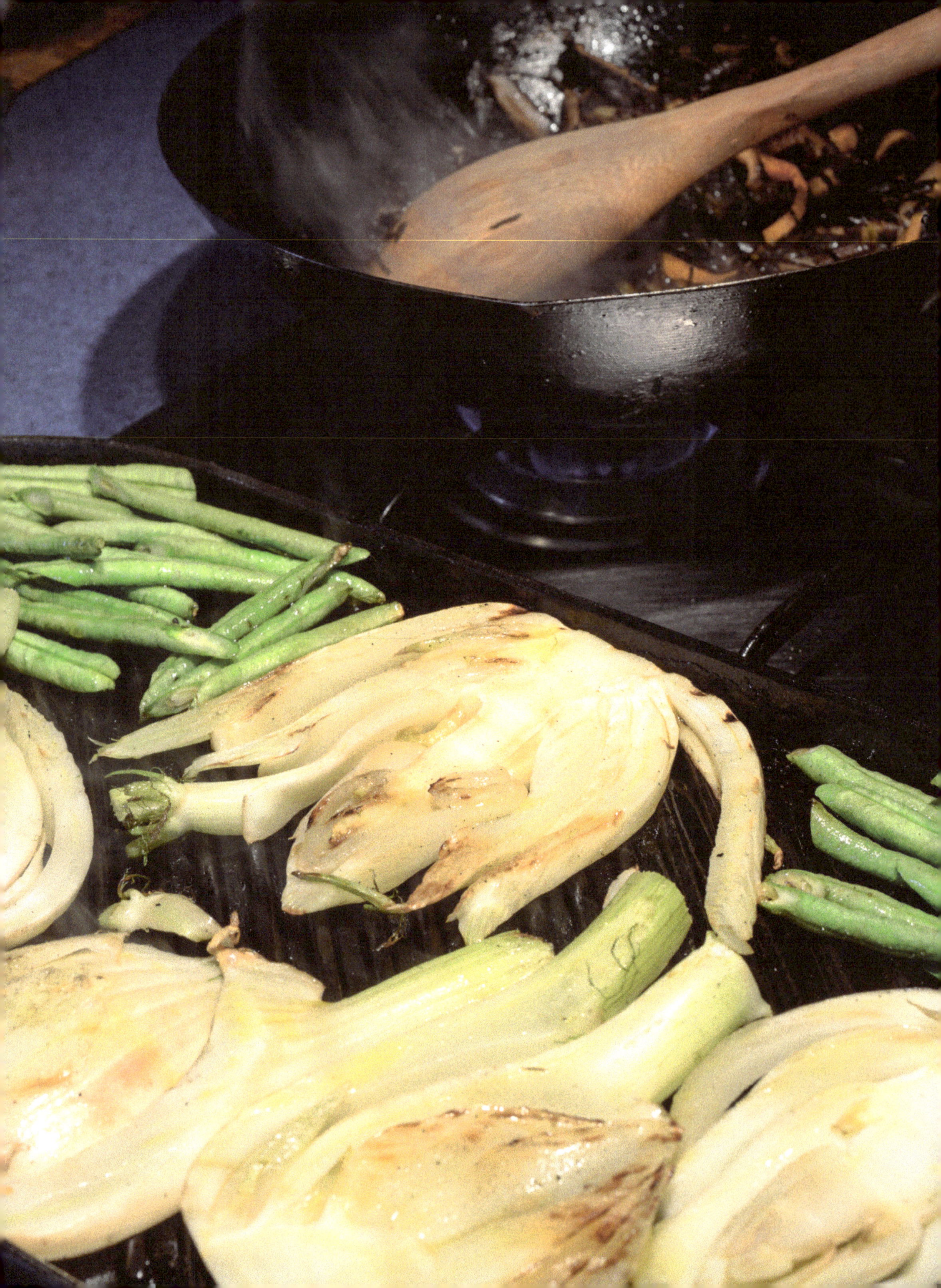

Lots More Vegetables

Kale Chips 66

Baked Beetroot, Grilled Snake Bean & Fennel 69

Vegetable Noodle (Voodle) Stir Fry 71

Baked Vegetable Noodles (Voodles) 73

Zucchini Pancakes 75

Broccoli Pancakes 77

Kale Almond Pancakes 77

KALE CHIPS

1 bunch	Kale
1 clove	Garlic, minced
1 tbsp	Extra virgin olive oil
1 tsp	Coconut syrup
¼ tsp	Sea salt

- Pre-heat oven to 120°C and line a tray with baking paper.
- Remove tough stalks from kale and tear leaves into pieces. Rinse and dry. Make sure kale pieces are really dry.
- In a bowl, mix minced garlic with olive oil, coconut syrup and salt.
- Place dry kale pieces in a large bowl and add half the dressing, then mix well with your hands. Depending on the quantity of kale, you can add more dressing if needed.
- Spread coated kale onto the tray and bake for about 15 to 20 minutes. Keep your eye on it and turn at least once. Bake until crisp but not brown. Remove from oven.
- Cool and eat immediately.

TIP: Storing homemade kale chips in containers, even glass containers, will cause them to become moist. To crisp up again, place in a pre-heated oven for a few minutes before serving.

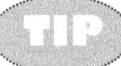

COOKING WITH KALE

There are many different types of kale. The leaves can be green or purple in colour, and have either a smooth or curly shape. Choose richly coloured, relatively small bunches of kale, and not any with limp or yellowing leaves.

Store kale in the coolest section of the refrigerator for no more than 2 or 3 days, as after that the flavour becomes quite strong and the leaves become limp.

Here is one of the favourite kale chips recipes, as enjoyed by all who have eaten them in my classes. I like these a little sweet to balance out the bitter flavour of the kale.

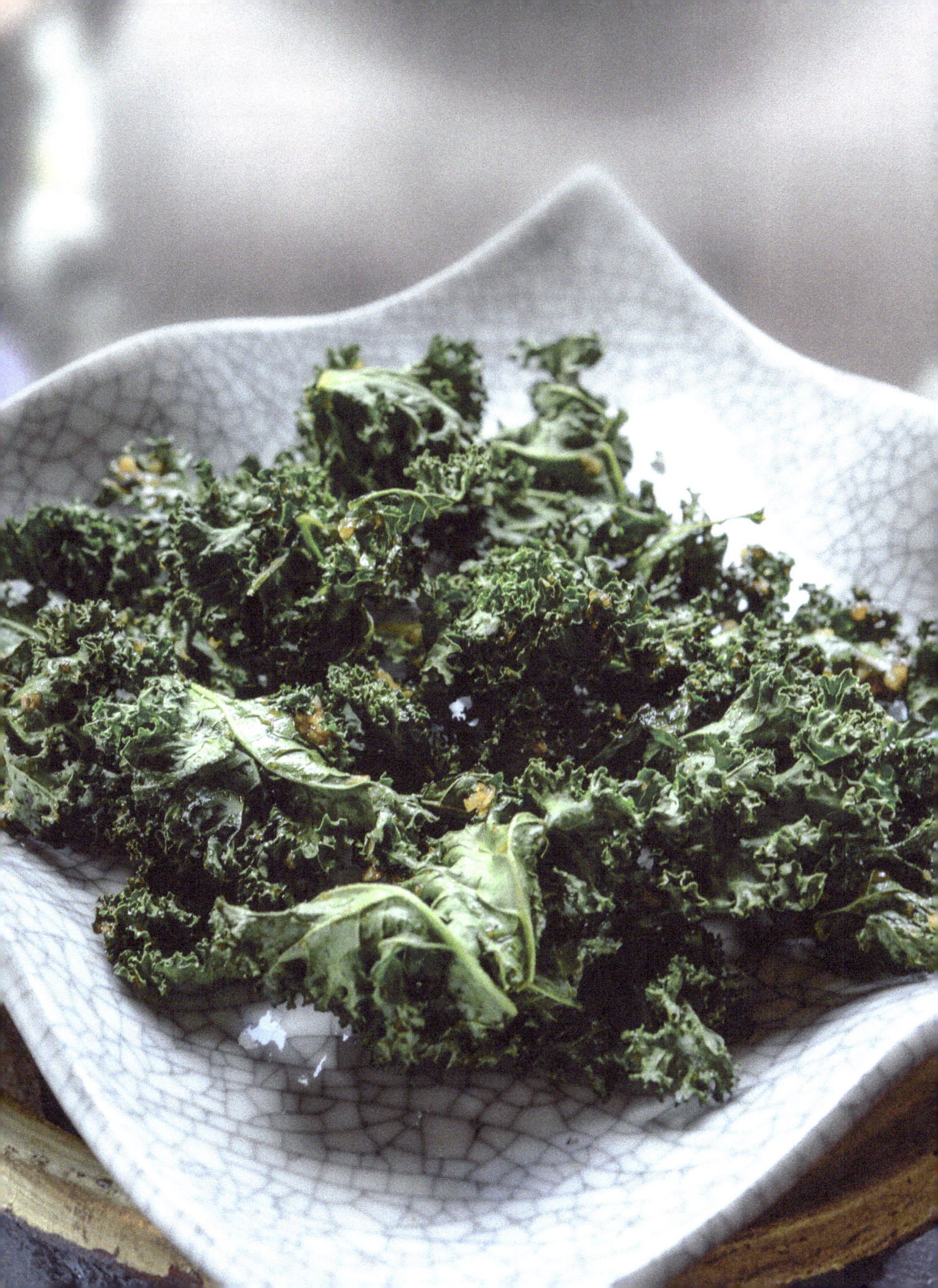

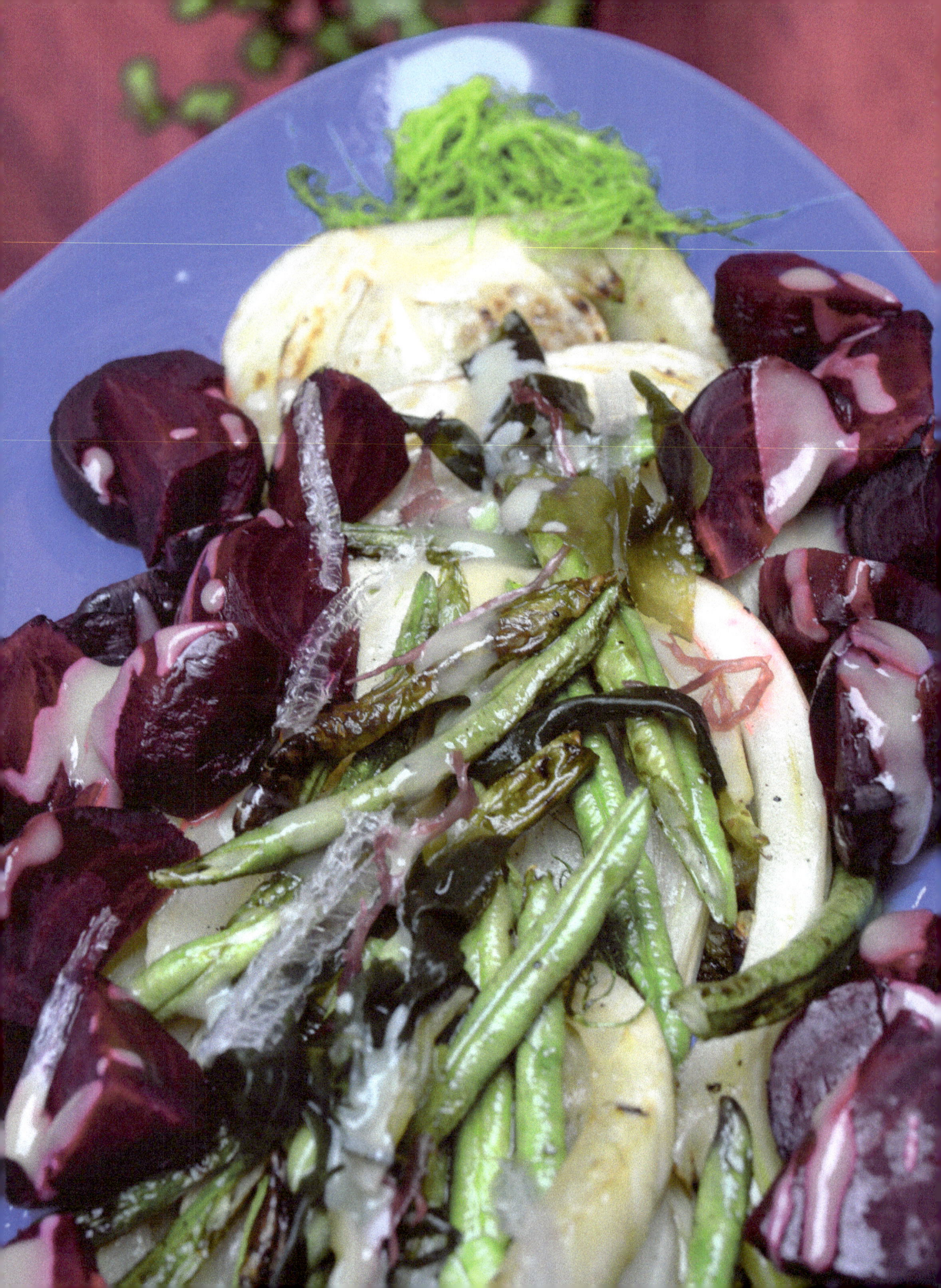

BAKED BEETROOT, GRILLED SNAKE BEAN & FENNEL
With Sweet Tahini Apple Cider Dressing

SERVES 4
KEEP REFRIGERATED. BEST USED WITHIN 3 DAYS

6 small	Beetroots
2 tbsp	Sea vegetable salad mix (Muso/Spiral Foods) (optional)
2 tbsp	Extra virgin olive oil
6	Snake beans or asparagus
1 medium	Fennel bulb (with tips)
30 g	Toasted walnuts
To taste	Sea salt and black pepper

SWEET TAHINI APPLE CIDER DRESSING

⅓ cup	Apple cider vinegar
2 tbsp	Rice syrup
2 tbsp	Tahini

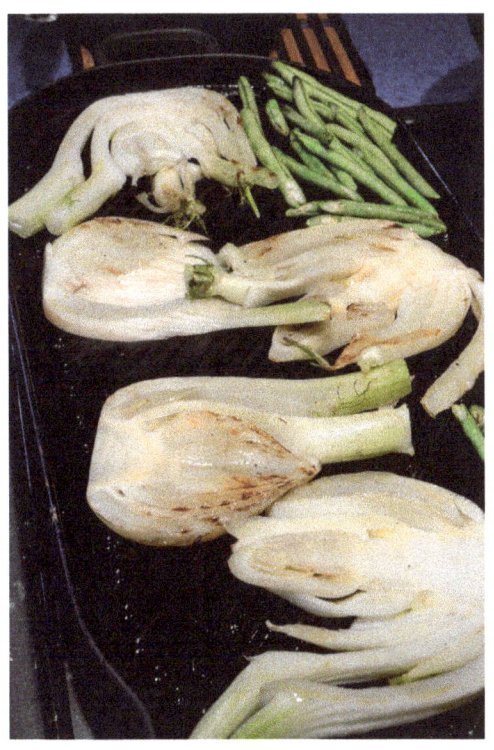

- Pre-heat oven to 200°C.
- Remove leaves and stems from beetroots – leaving a little at the top of each beetroot – and wash well.
- Place in ovenproof dish and cover with foil to bake for about 45 minutes or until beetroots are cooked. You can add a little water to the dish to create more steam.
- Remove from oven and cool. If you prefer, peel cooked beetroots (I like keeping the skin on, especially if the beetroots are organic) then cut into eighths. Set aside.
- In a small bowl, mix ingredients for dressing.
- Soak sea vegetable salad mix for 5 to 10 minutes in water to cover. Drain.
- If using snake beans, wash and cut into 8 cm lengths. If using thick asparagus, make shavings with a potato peeler. If using thin asparagus, then use as is.
- Remove any tough or brown outer layers of fennel and cut in half. Remove a little of the hard root, slice the rest into ½ cm strips and keep leafy tops for garnish. (If you use a mandolin, place fennel cut side down and shave into thin slices.)
- Pour oil into a cast iron griddle (using one with raised griddle ridges looks good) and sear fennel and beans for about 2 minutes on one side then turn and cook for a further minute. Remove from pan to cool.
- Place all vegetables on a serving plate and add chopped toasted walnuts and drizzle on dressing.
- Garnish with fennel tips.

When in season, use asparagus instead of snake beans.

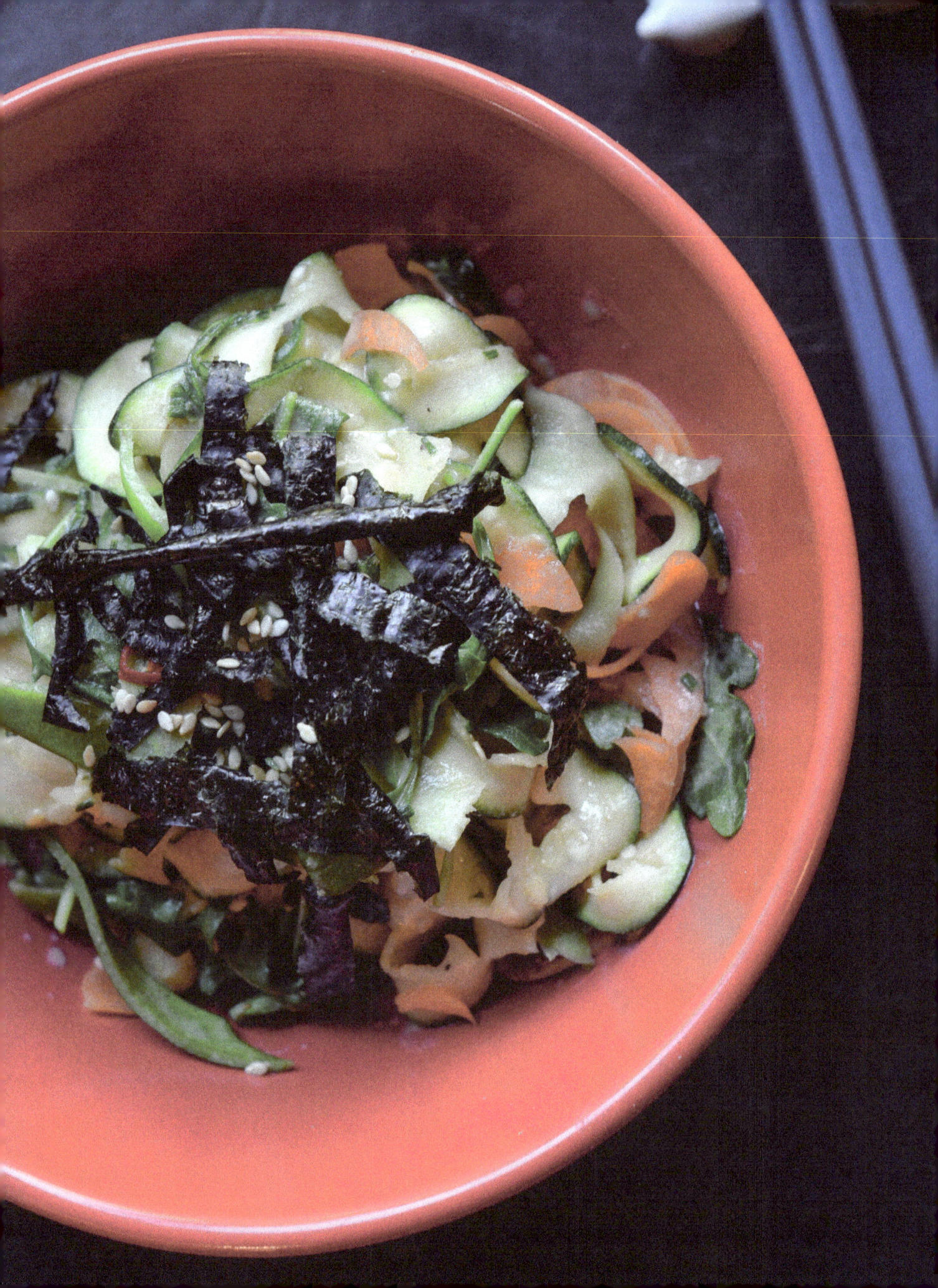

VEGETABLE NOODLE (VOODLE) STIR FRY
With White Miso Sauce

SERVES 4

1 stem	Broccoli (cut stem from 1 head of broccoli)
1	Carrot
1	Zucchini
6	Snow peas
1–2	Red chilli, to taste
4 tbsp	White miso paste (Shiro)
2 tbsp	Tahini
2 tbsp	Lemon or lime juice
2 tbsp	Mirin (optional)
½ cup	Water
1 tbsp	Toasted sesame oil
2	Garlic cloves, minced, to taste
1 tbsp	Ginger, grated
6	Chives, chopped, to taste
1–2 cups	Watercress or rocket (arugula), as required
Pinch	Black pepper
1 tbsp	Toasted sesame seeds
Garnish	Dulse flakes or shredded sushi nori

- Peel off and trim away any tough parts of the broccoli stem but keep the leafy bits to add to the mix.
- Use a peeler or spiraliser to shave long strips from the broccoli stem, carrot and zucchini.
- Slice snow peas and chilli into thin strips.
- In a bowl, mix miso, tahini, lemon or lime juice and mirin (if using) with water.
- Heat sesame oil in wok. Add garlic and ginger and fry for about 30 seconds.
- Add broccoli, carrot, zucchini, snow peas and chilli and fry over high heat.
- Add miso mix and more water if needed.
- Add chives, watercress or rocket, black pepper and toss gently to heat through.
- Sprinkle with toasted sesame seeds.
- Garnish with dulse flakes or sushi nori strips to serve.

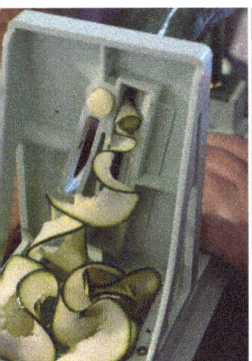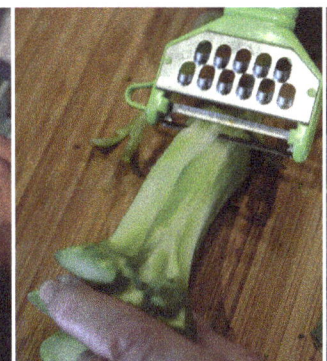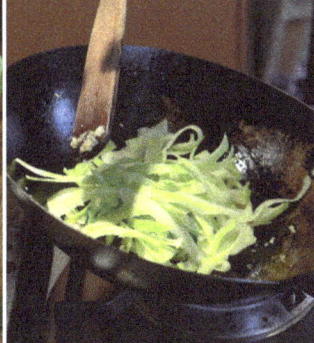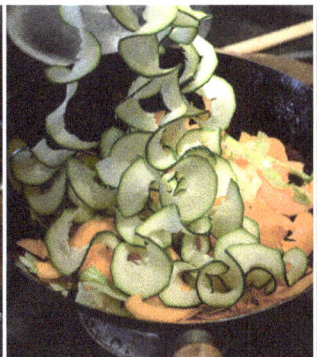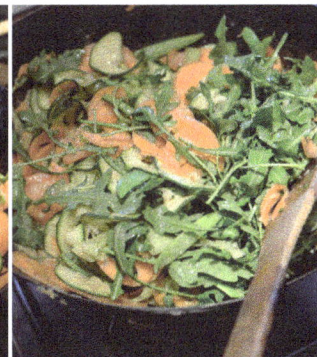

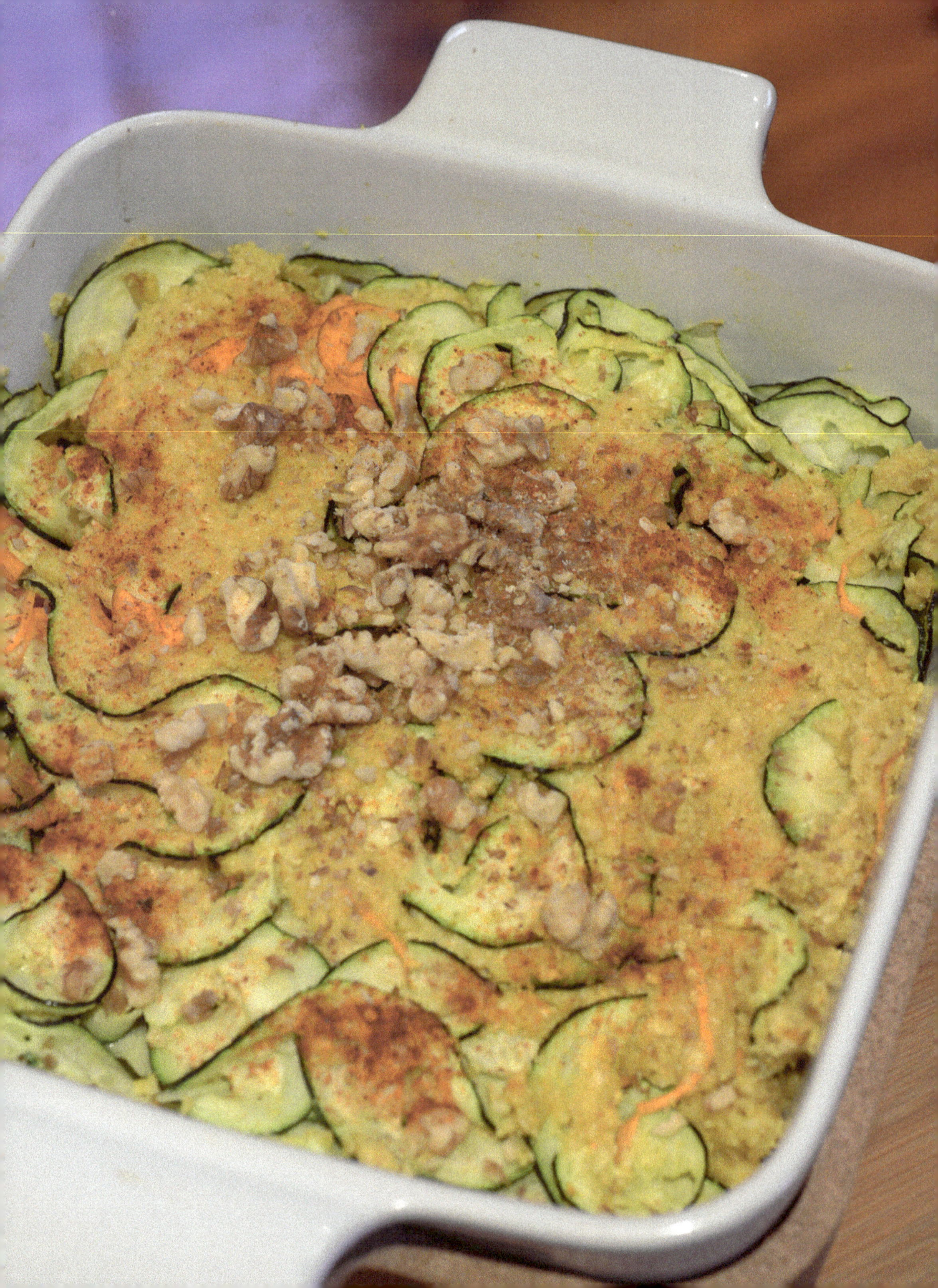

BAKED VEGETABLE NOODLES (VOODLES)
With Cashew 'Cheese' Sauce

SERVES 4–6
ONCE COOLED, KEEP LEFTOVERS, REFRIGERATED,
FOR UP TO 3 DAYS

4 medium	Zucchini
2 medium	Carrots
Pinch	Sea salt
As required	Walnuts, finely chopped
As required	Chilli or cayenne pepper, to taste
Garnish	Basil, chopped

CASHEW 'CHEESE' SAUCE

2 cups	Cashews
2 tbsp	Lemon juice
2 tbsp	Water
½ cup	Extra virgin olive oil
1 clove	Garlic, minced
¼–½	Shallot, to taste
1 tsp	Sea salt
¼ cup	Savoury yeast flakes
½–1 tsp	Chilli powder or flakes
Pinch	Cayenne pepper
Pinch	Turmeric, ground or fresh, grated
Pinch	Black pepper

- Process zucchini and carrots though a spiral slicer or spiraliser to create noodles or use a wide blade peeler. Toss with a bit of sea salt and let sit for 30 minutes.
- Pre-heat oven to 120°C.
- Make cashew 'cheese' sauce (recipe below).
- Mix voodles and cashew 'cheese' sauce in a bowl then spread into a casserole pan.
- Top with finely chopped walnuts and sprinkle with extra chilli or cayenne to your taste.
- Place casserole pan in bottom of pre-heated oven for 20 to 30 minutes or until warm.
- Garnish with chopped basil before serving.

THE SAUCE

- Soak cashews for 2 hours, then rinse and drain.
- Blend all ingredients in food processor or blender until completely smooth. Add a little water if required. Adjust seasonings to taste.

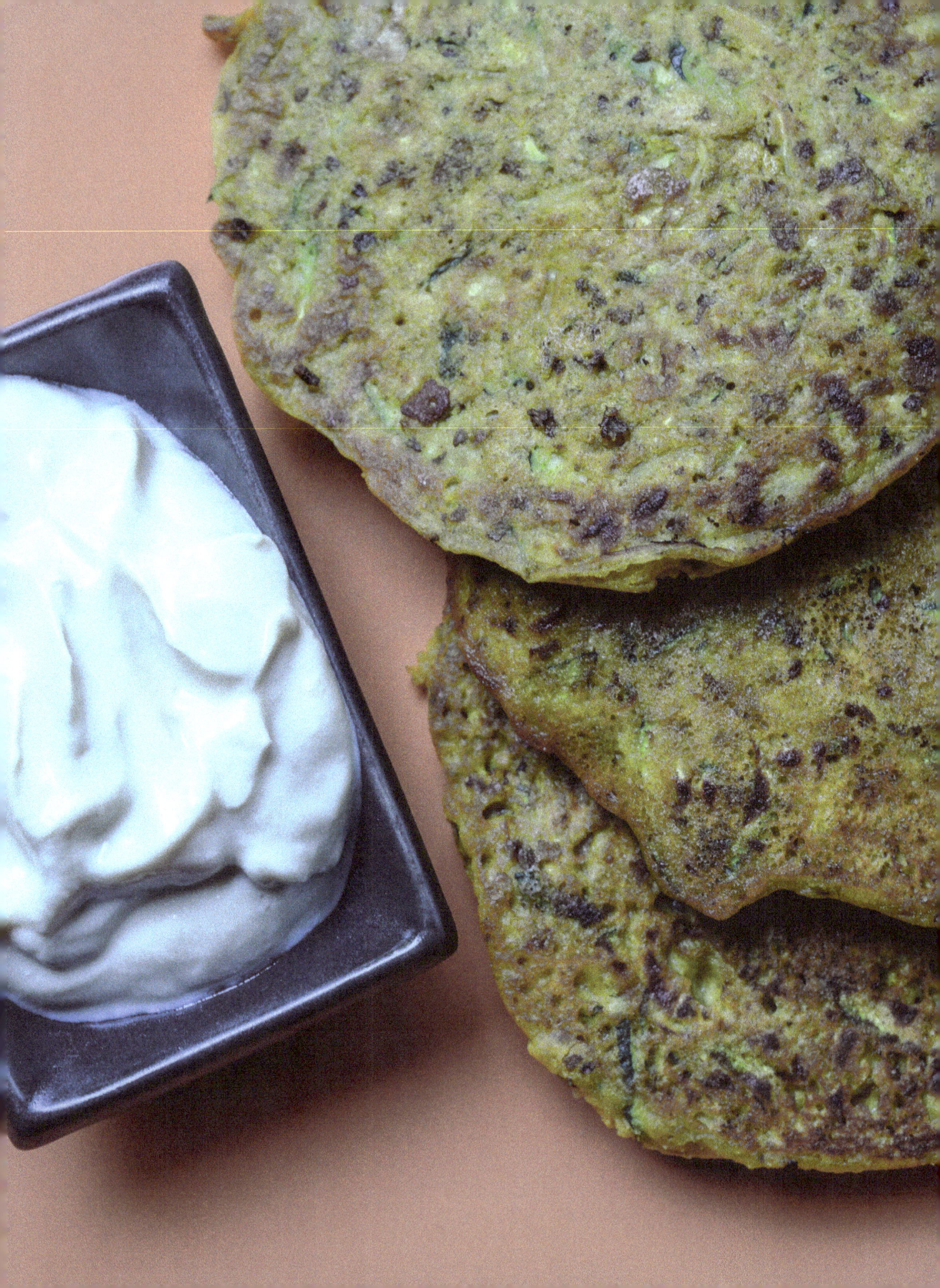

ZUCCHINI PANCAKES
With Tofu Sour Cream

MAKES 6 X 8 CM PANCAKES
LEFTOVERS CAN BE STORED IN AN AIRTIGHT CONTAINER IN THE REFRIGERATOR FOR UP TO 3 DAYS

1 cup	Chickpea (besan) flour
1 large	Zucchini, grated
⅓ cup	Spring onion, sliced, or fennel, finely diced
½–1 tsp	Cumin, ground
½ tsp	Cayenne pepper
½ tsp	Turmeric, ground or 1 tsp fresh, grated
2 tbsp	Dulse flakes
½ tsp	Sea salt
½ cup	Water
	Coconut oil

TOFU SOUR CREAM
MAKES 1 ½ CUPS
KEEPS REFRIGERATED FOR UP TO 5 DAYS

325 g	Silken tofu
1 tbsp	Extra virgin olive oil
4 tbsp	Fresh lemon juice
2 tbsp	Apple cider vinegar
2 tsp	Liquid sweetener of your choice, e.g. rice syrup
½ tsp	Sea salt

- Mix grated zucchini into flour, adding spring onion or fennel, spices, dulse flakes, sea salt and water until combined.
- Allow the mixture to rest for 10 minutes to absorb the water.
- Heat coconut oil in a flat skillet and, when hot, add a large spoonful of mixture (to make an 8 cm pancake). Cook until bubbles form on surface and flip over to cook until pancake is cooked through and golden brown.
- Place cooked pancake on a plate and cover with baking paper or another plate to keep warm while you repeat the process with remaining mixture.
- Serve with any Dip : Dress : Spread : Top recipe or this delicious tofu sour cream.

THE CREAM
- Place all ingredients in a blender. Process for several minutes, until very creamy and smooth.
- Serve on baked or steamed vegetables, soups or pancakes.

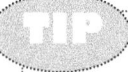

FLIPPING PANCAKES

Don't touch them with a spatula after you've poured them into the pan. As soon as you see lots of air bubbles rising to the top, you can test the edges. Then if they feel solid, carefully pry your spatula underneath the pancake, and flip!

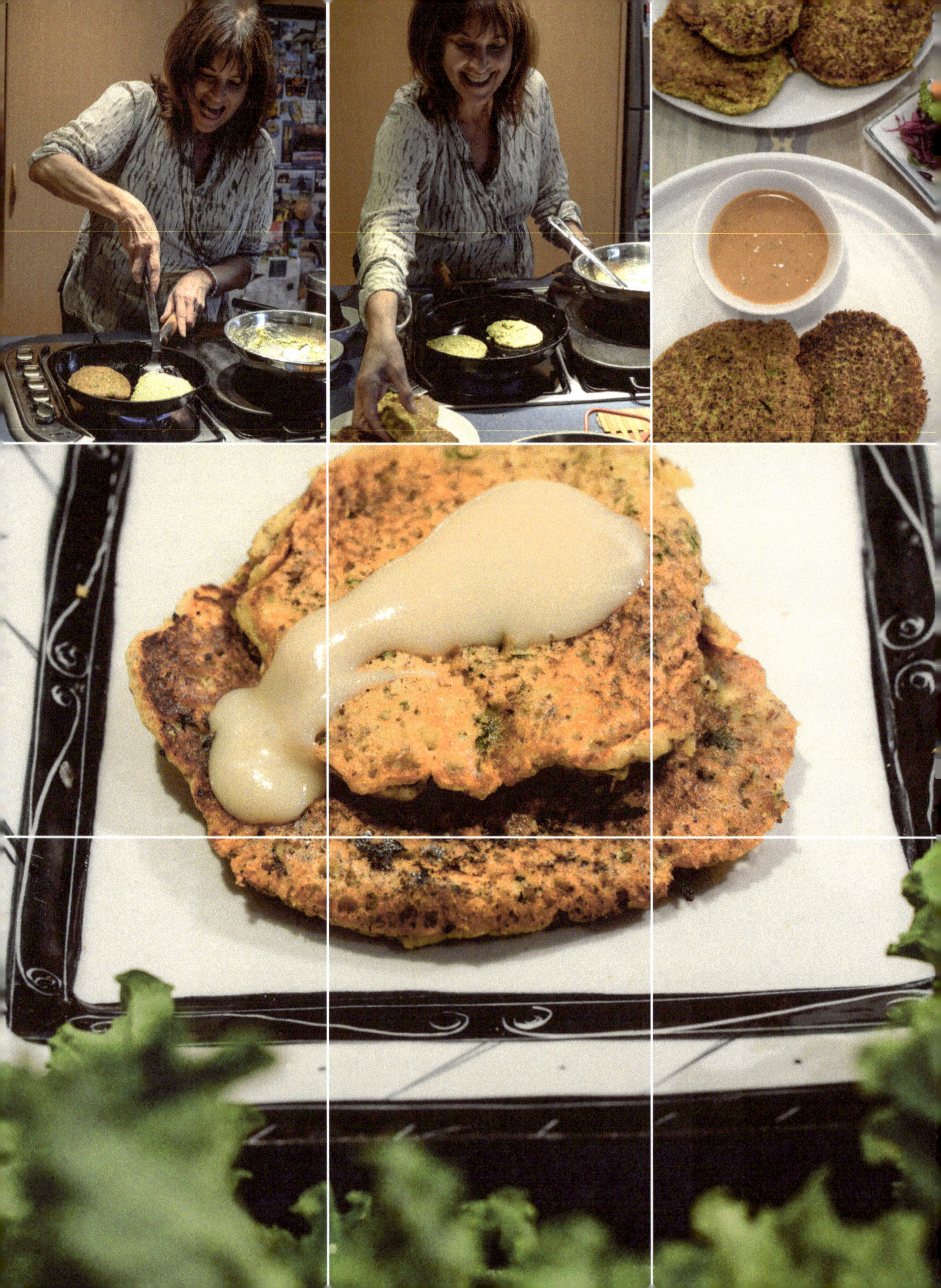

Flaxegg is a great egg substitute — see glossary for more information.

BROCCOLI PANCAKES

MAKES ABOUT 8 X 8 CM PANCAKES
LEFTOVERS CAN BE STORED IN AN AIRTIGHT
CONTAINER IN THE REFRIGERATOR FOR UP TO 3 DAYS

⅔ cup	Chickpea (besan) flour
½ cup	Buckwheat flour
½–1 tsp	Sea salt, to taste
2 tsp	Baking powder (use gluten-free if required)
2 tbsp	Flaxseeds, ground
6 tbsp	Water (to soak ground flaxseeds)
2 cups	Broccoli florets, chopped
2–3 cloves	Garlic, sliced
1 small	Chilli, sliced or 1 tsp chilli paste
1 tsp	Cumin, ground
1 tsp	Coriander, ground
1 tsp	Turmeric, ground
1¼ cups	Water
3–4 tsp	Sesame oil

- Mix flours, salt and baking powder in a large bowl.
- Prepare flaxegg: mix the flax seeds with the 6 tbsp of water and set aside.
- Place chopped broccoli, sliced garlic and chilli, spices and remaining water into a high-speed blender or food processor and blend until smooth.
- Pour mixture into dry ingredients and add flaxegg. Mix well by hand or with a spoon to make a smooth batter. Set aside for 5 minutes.
- Heat frypan with oil and, when hot, spoon in ¼ cup (4 tbsp) of mixture. Cook until bubbles form on surface and flip over to cook until pancake is cooked through and golden brown (see tip on previous page).
- Place cooked pancake on a plate and cover with baking paper or another plate to keep warm while you repeat the process with remaining mixture.
- Serve with any Dip : Dress : Spread : Top recipe. A big favourite is the creamy ginger sauce.

KALE ALMOND PANCAKES

MAKES ABOUT 8 X 8 CM PANCAKES
LEFTOVERS CAN BE STORED IN AN AIRTIGHT
CONTAINER IN THE REFRIGERATOR FOR UP TO 3 DAYS

⅔ cup	Chickpea (besan) flour
½ cup	Almonds, ground
Pinch	Sea salt, to taste
1 tsp	Baking powder (use gluten-free if required)
1 tbsp	Chia seeds
1 tbsp	Maple syrup or any liquid sweetener
1 tsp	Ras el hanout (or ground coriander or chilli)
1 cup	Kale, finely chopped, pressed into cup
1¼ cups	Almond Mylk (see Nut Mylk p132)
1 tbsp	Flaxseeds, ground
3 tbsp	Water (to soak ground flaxseeds)

- Prepare flaxegg: mix the flax seeds with the 6 tbsp of water and set aside.
- Mix together chickpea flour, ground almonds, salt, baking powder, chia seeds and spices.
- Place almond mylk, kale and maple syrup in a high-speed blender and blend until smooth.
- Pour this mixture, along with the flaxegg, into the dry ingredients, and mix to form a smooth batter. Set aside for 5 minutes.
- Heat frypan with oil and, when hot, spoon in ¼ cup (4 tbsp) of mixture. Cook until bubbles form on surface and flip over to cook until pancake is cooked through and golden brown (see tip on previous page).
- Place cooked pancake on a plate and cover with baking paper or another plate to keep warm while you repeat the process with remaining mixture.
- Serve with any Dip : Dress : Spread : Top recipe. I used miso tahini lemon sauce for the photo. Try tofu sour cream too.

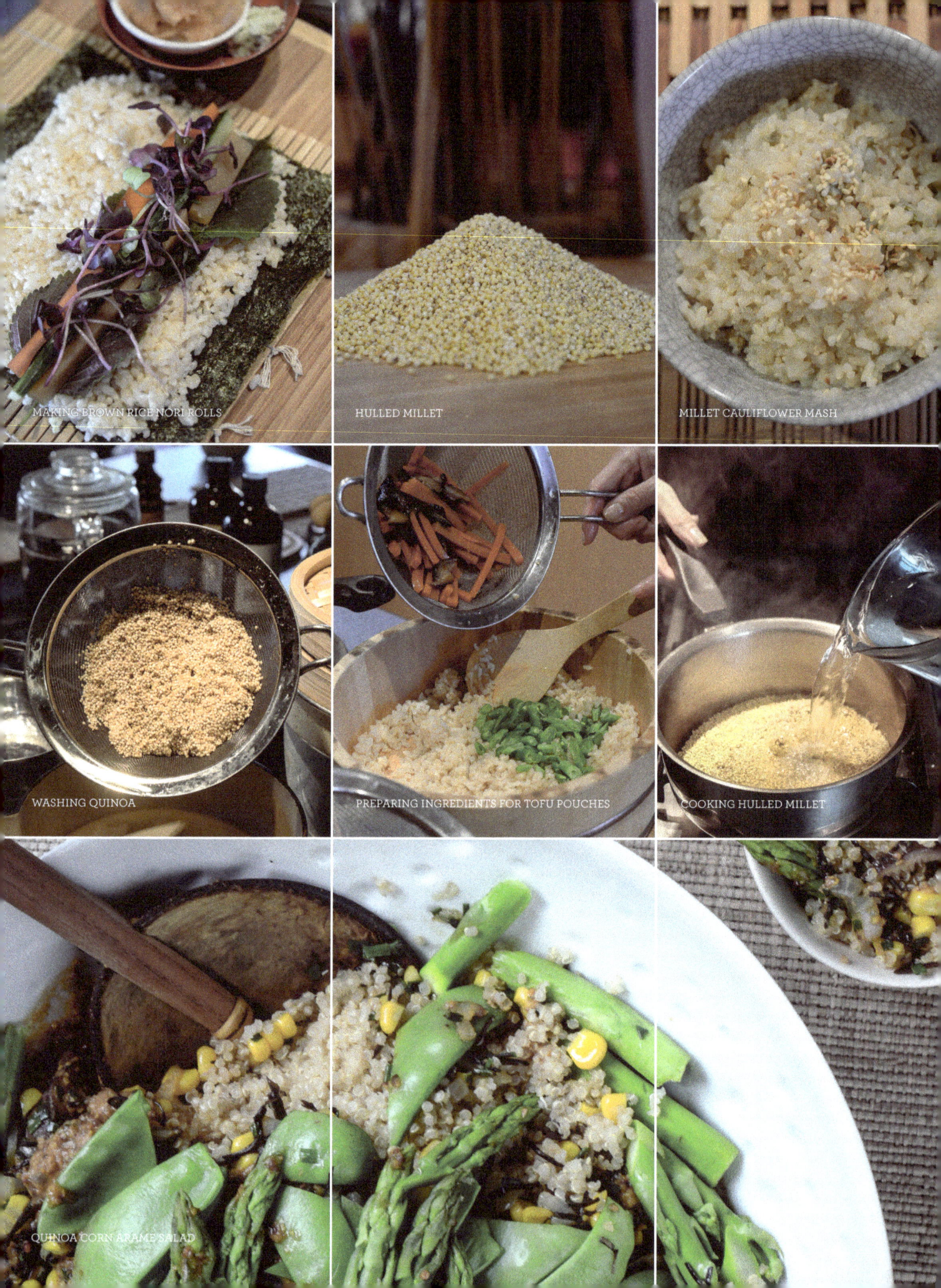

MAKING BROWN RICE NORI ROLLS

HULLED MILLET

MILLET CAULIFLOWER MASH

WASHING QUINOA

PREPARING INGREDIENTS FOR TOFU POUCHES

COOKING HULLED MILLET

QUINOA CORN ARAME SALAD

Essential Wholegrains

Cooking Hulled Millet 80

Millet Cauliflower Mash 80

Pumpkin Millet Seed Balls 81

Cooking Brown Rice 82

Sea Vegetable Brown Rice 82

Brown Rice For Sushi 83

Tofu Pouches – Inari Sushi 85

Brown Rice Vegetable Paella 87

Quinoa Black Bean Patties 89

Quinoa Corn Arame Salad 91

Buckwheat Chickpea Tabbouleh 93

COOKING HULLED MILLET

MAKES ABOUT 3 CUPS

This is my favourite wholegrain. Since it is a small grain, millet does not require soaking. Pan-toasting before cooking will give you a nuttier flavour.

1 cup	Hulled millet
3 cups	Water
Pinch	Sea salt

- Wash millet and drain well. Toast millet slowly in a dry saucepan for several minutes until fragrant and you hear some popping sounds. Remove into a bowl.
- In a saucepan, bring water to a boil, add toasted millet and, when the pot returns to the boil, add a pinch of sea salt.
- Cover with the lid, turn heat to low (use a heat diffuser if you have one) and simmer for about 25 minutes or until millet has absorbed the water. (You can peek in, but don't stir.)
- Remove from heat and leave it to steam with the lid on for a further 10 minutes before serving.

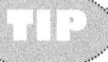# MILLET VARIATIONS

1 cup dry hulled millet = about 3 cups cooked.

In general, use water to grain ratio of 3:1. For millet porridge you can use up to 5:1 and for pilaf and baked millet dishes use 2:1.

If using a higher proportion of water, you may cook millet longer until the grain becomes very soft.

Add 1–2 pinches of sea salt per cup of grain.

MILLET CAULIFLOWER MASH

SERVES 4-5

1 tsp	Toasted sesame oil
1 cup	Hulled millet
1 ½ cups	Cauliflower florets
1 tsp	Turmeric, fresh, grated or ½ tsp ground
Pinch	Sea salt
3 ½ cups	Water
Garnish	Sesame sea vegetable seasoning

- Wash and drain millet.
- Heat oil in a saucepan. Add millet and sauté for 3 minutes.
- Add cauliflower florets, turmeric, sea salt and water. Bring to a boil.
- Reduce heat and simmer, covered, for 30 minutes. Use a heat diffuser if you have one. (Don't stir to ensure steam cooks millet evenly.)
- Remove from heat and leave it to steam with the lid on for a further 15 minutes.
- Mash and serve.

I like to eat this with miso tahini lemon sauce.

PUMPKIN MILLET SEED BALLS

MAKES ABOUT 15 BALLS (DEPENDING ON HOW BIG YOU MAKE THEM)

1 cup	Hulled millet, rinsed and drained
1 cup	Pumpkin, skin removed and cut into 2 cm cubes
2 ½ cups	Water
Pinch	Sea salt
½ cup	Sandy's seed mix (see recipe p.124)
1 tbsp	Tahini (I prefer hulled tahini)
1–2 tsp	Tamari or shoyu, to taste
Garnish	Dulse flakes

- Pour water into a medium saucepan and bring to a boil.
- Add hulled millet, cubed pumpkin and a pinch of sea salt. Cover and simmer gently for 25 minutes. (Use a heat diffuser if you have one.)
- Turn off the heat, take the lid off and let cool for about 5 minutes before mashing the mixture.
- Once it has cooled even further, place mixture into a bowl and add the seeds, tahini and tamari or shoyu. Mix well.
- Using your hands, roll a small amount of millet mix to make into bite-sized balls.

You can also serve this as a mash.

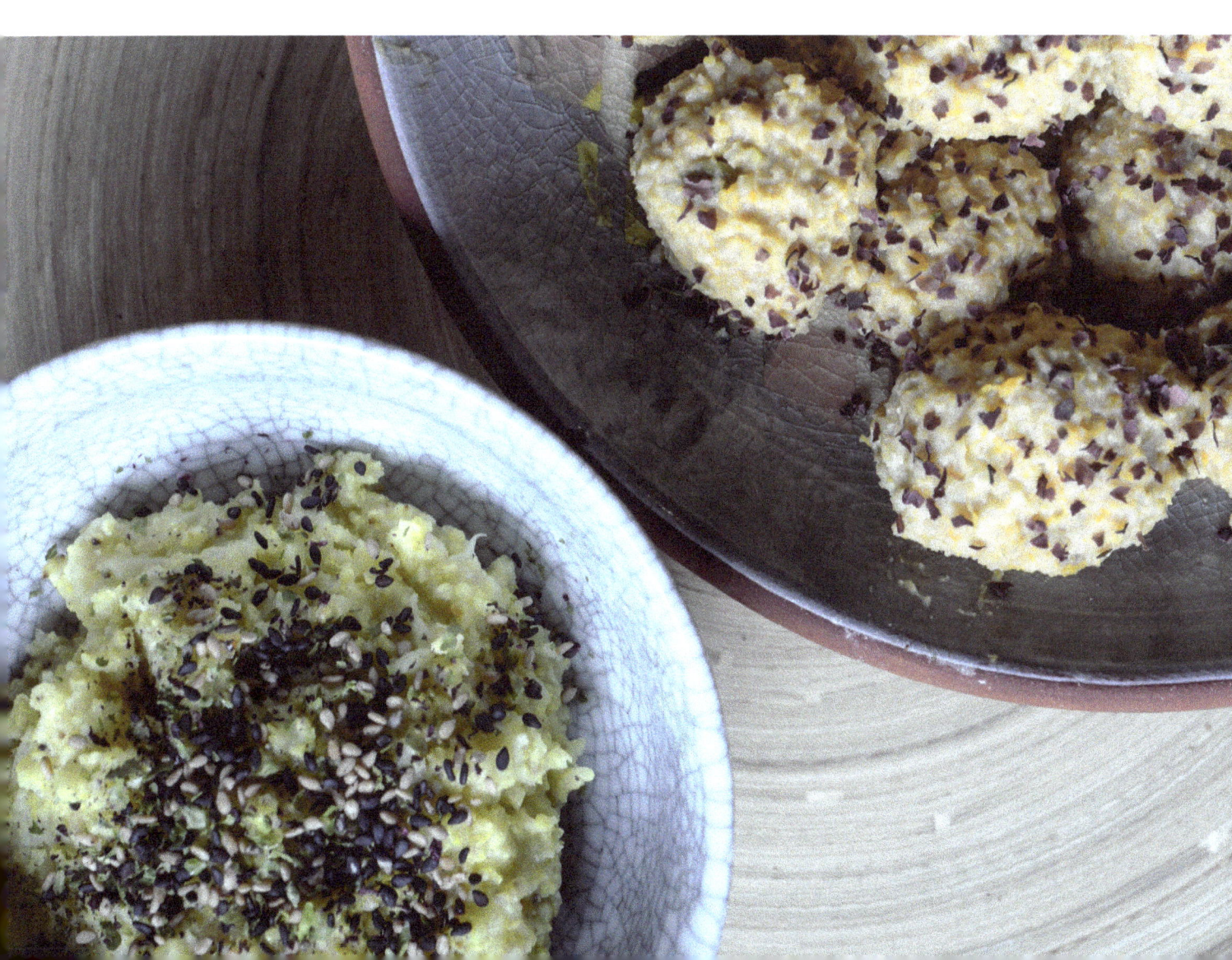

COOKING BROWN RICE

MAKES ABOUT 2 ½ CUPS

1 cup	Brown rice (use biodynamic rice if you can)
2.2 cups	Water
Pinch	Sea salt

Use leftover brown rice to make brown rice porridge (p150).

- Soak rice for at least 30 minutes, though 3 hours or even all day is best.
- Wash rice, drain and place in saucepan with water and sea salt.
- Bring to a boil over a high heat without the lid. When the rice boils, cover it and simmer slowly for 30 minutes. Don't stir.
- Turn off the heat and leave it to steam with the lid on for further 10 minutes.

My comfort food

SEA VEGETABLE BROWN RICE

SERVES 4

1 cup	Brown rice (shorter grain makes stickier rice, which is what I prefer)
5 cm	Wakame
½ medium	Onion, minced
2 cloves	Garlic, minced
2 tbsp	Sesame seeds, toasted (see tip on p.40)
Pinch	Sea salt and black pepper

- Soak rice for at least 30 minutes, though 3 hours or even all day is best. Rinse and drain. (For soaking health benefits, see glossary p.154)
- Soak wakame in 2¼ cups of water for 5 minutes, remove stem and chop. Retain soaking water.
- Heat 1 tbsp of wakame soaking water in a medium to heavy-based saucepan.
- Sauté onion over medium heat for 1 minute. Stir in garlic, rice, chopped wakame, toasted sesame seeds and rest of wakame soaking water.
- Bring to a boil over high heat. Don't stir.
- As soon as it begins to boil, reduce heat to low and cover. Simmer for 35 minutes. Don't stir.
- Turn off the heat and leave it to steam for another 10 minutes.
- Season with sea salt and pepper to taste and serve.

BROWN RICE FOR SUSHI

1 cup	Short grain brown rice
2 ¼ cups	Water
2 tsp	Tamari or shoyu

SUSHI VINEGAR MIX

3 tbsp	Brown rice vinegar
2 tbsp	White sugar (we do use sugar for this traditional method) or use your preferred sweetener
1 tbsp	Sea salt
6 cm	Kombu (optional)

Use this rice for my sushi rolls (norimaki), nori pyramids (onigiri) and tofu pouches (inari sushi).

- Wash rice in cold water, stir and wash away floating husks. Wash several times until the rinsing water is clear, then place rice in a saucepan and add measured water and tamari or shoyu.
- Soak for at least 30 minutes.
- Bring to boil then cover and lower heat to simmer for 30 minutes or until all the water has been absorbed. Don't stir.
- Turn off the heat and leave it to steam with lid on for another 10 minutes.
- Place vinegar, sugar, sea salt and kombu (if using) in a small saucepan and simmer gently until sugar is dissolved. If using kombu, remove from mixture before using vinegar mixture to make sushi rice.
- Place cooked rice in a hangiri wooden sushi rice bowl, or, if you don't have one, a glass bowl (don't use plastic) and slowly add the vinegar mixture.
- Cool the rice by lightly tossing in the vinegar mix until it reaches room temperature. Don't put the rice in the refrigerator to make it cool faster as that will damage the rice. You can, however, use a fan as you toss.
- Cover with a clean damp cloth until you're ready to use it – use within 2 hours.

TIP — SUSHI RICE

It's best not to store cooked sushi rice in the refrigerator as it loses flavour and becomes dry and hard to eat. For proper hygiene and the best-tasting sushi, always make fresh sushi rice and use promptly.

VARIATION: Use a natural ready-made sushi vinegar instead of making your own. I recommend Spiral Foods sushi vinegar.
For a tasty different flavour, you can use Japanese plum vinegar (Ume Su) instead of brown rice vinegar.

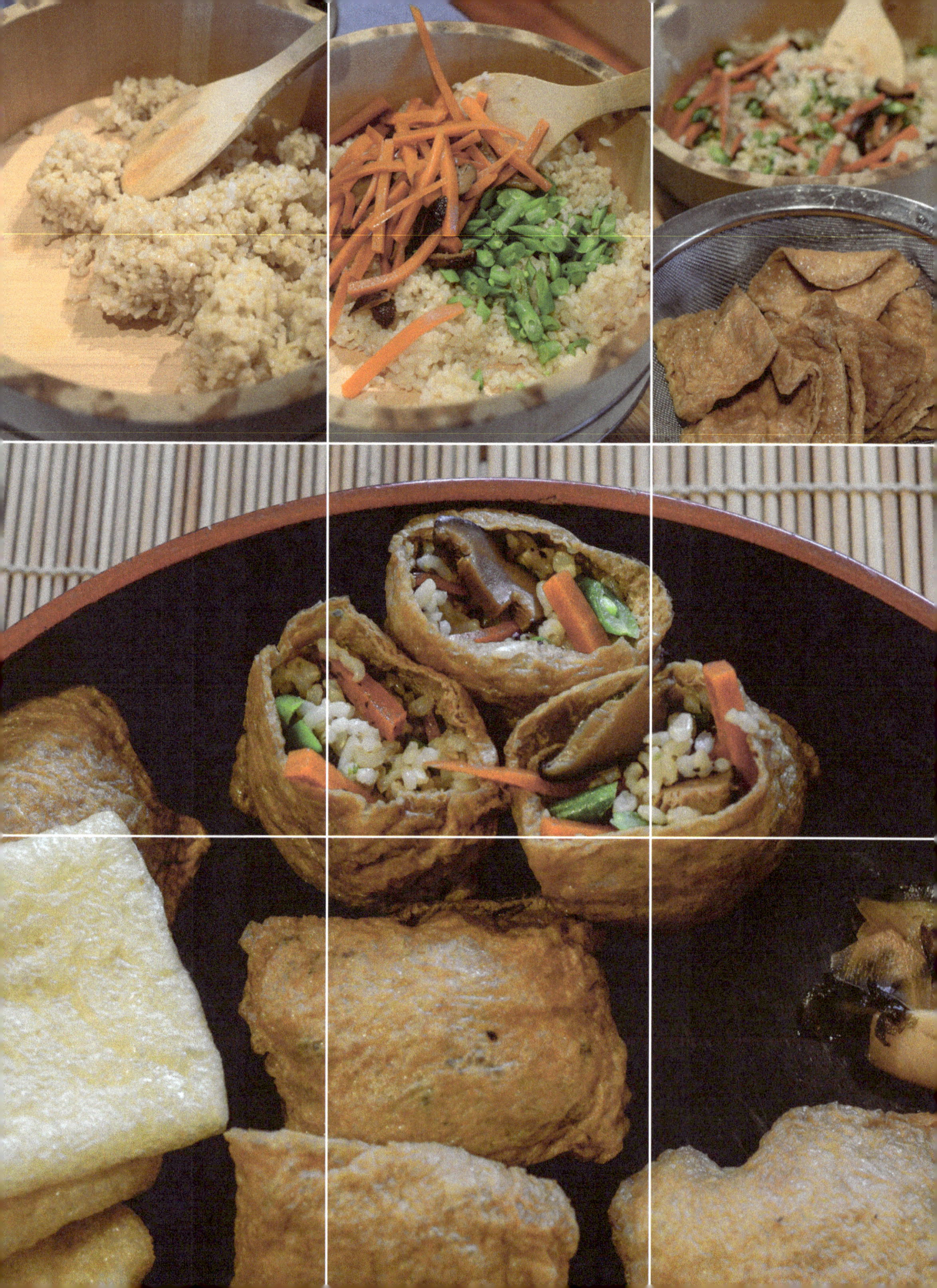

TOFU POUCHES – INARI SUSHI

MAKES 12 POUCHES

1 quantity	Cooked brown sushi rice (see recipe)
4	Shiitake, dried
¼	Carrot, julienned
2 packets	Fried bean curd (can be found in frozen section of Japanese supermarkets. Also called abura age)
¼ cup	Mirin
¼ cup	Tamari
1 cup	Dashi stock (use a sachet) or shiitake soaking water stock
1 tbsp	Honey or any liquid sweetener of your choice
4	String beans
3 tbsp	Pickled ginger, to taste
pinch	Sea salt
1–2 tbsp	Toasted sesame seeds

- Soak shiitake mushrooms for at least 30 minutes in 1½ cups warm water from the kettle or for even better flavour, soak overnight.
- When mushrooms have softened, discard stems then slice mushrooms caps. Strain shiitake soaking water and keep to use as stock.
- Place carrot, sliced shiitake and tofu pouches in a small saucepan with mirin, tamari, dashi stock or shiitake soaking water and sweetener and simmer for approximately 15 minutes. Cool.
- Thinly slice string beans on the diagonal then blanch in salted boiling water for 1 minute. Drain.
- Mix chopped pickled ginger, string beans, shiitake, carrot and sesame seeds into cooked sushi rice and stuff into cooled marinated tofu pouches.

Folklore: Inari is the Shinto god of rice and the harvest, and the fox, his messenger, is famous for his love of deep-fried tofu.

A golden pouch of sushi rice with vegetables in marinated bean curd – always popular!

I met Sandy when I came into her Soulfood/Manna Health Food Store in the 80's. I was already interested in natural foods and healthy lifestyle discovering that healthy mindful eating adds to my happiness. Cooking and eating Sandy's food always makes me feel elevated and suits my challenged digestive system. I have been to many of her cooking classes including repeats of classes, as I find them great reminders and of course I get to eat her delicious meals at the classes. Over the years I have also had one-on-one consultation to support my weak digestive system and help deal with inflammation. My favourite recipes include her Super Miso Soup, Broccoli pancakes and easy recipes using greens and sea vegetables.

What stays with me every day is the knowledge passed on by Sandy of soaking grains and especially chewing. I've learnt to keep a clean pantry i.e. shop day to day for fresh ingredients while keeping a few basic staples. It's people like Sandy, who are passionate about sharing healthy knowledge and who help to support our wellbeing.

Melma Hamersfeld, Melbourne

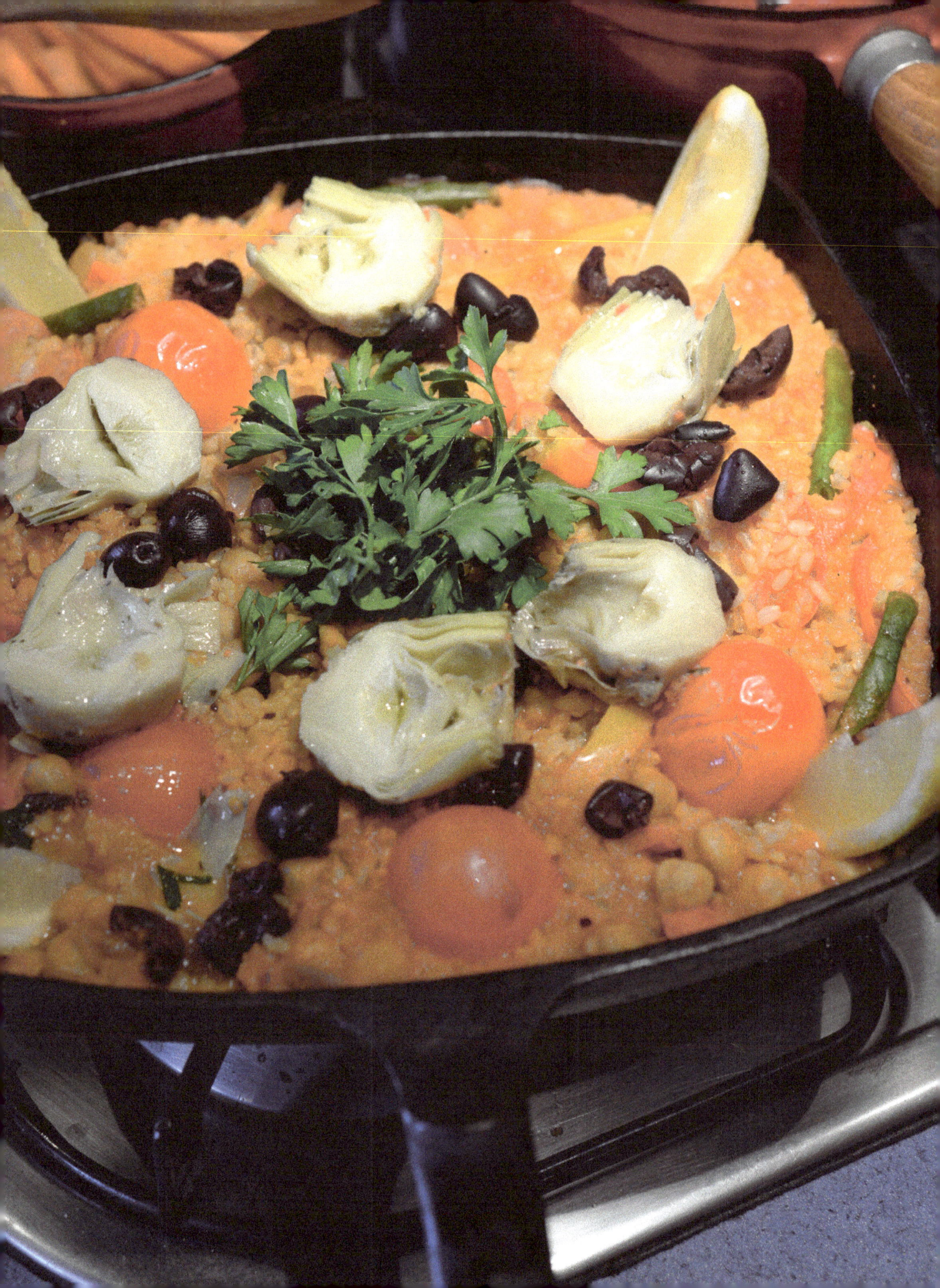

BROWN RICE VEGETABLE PAELLA

SERVES 4–6

1 cup	Short-grain brown rice
8 threads	Saffron
3 cups	Vegetable stock (see recipe p.16)
1 tbsp	Extra virgin olive oil
1 large	Red onion, diced
4 cloves	Garlic, thinly sliced
1 small	Red capsicum, sliced
1 small	Yellow capsicum, sliced
2 tbsp	Tomato paste
¾ cup	Cherry tomatoes, fresh, crushed or tinned crushed tomatoes
To taste	Sea salt and pepper
½ tbsp	Smoked paprika
1 cup	String beans, trimmed and halved
1 cup	Chickpeas, cooked or tinned
3	Artichoke hearts, sliced (can be freshly cooked, frozen or tinned)
10–15	Black olives, pitted
Garnish	Lemon wedges
¼ cup	Parsley, chopped for garnish

This is great served in a traditional paella pan but if you don't have one, a large cast-iron or oven-proof skillet is fine.

- Soak short-grain brown rice in enough water to cover for at least 30 minutes. Drain.
- Bring 3 cups of water with a pinch of salt to a boil, add rice and cook for about 20 minutes, or until rice begins to soften. Drain and set aside. (Parboiling brown rice speeds up its overall cooking time.)
- Heat oven to 200°C.
- Combine saffron threads with 4 tbsp of warm water in a small bowl and set aside.
- In a large pot, bring vegetable stock to a simmer, then reduce the heat and keep at a low simmer until needed.
- Heat the olive oil in a large cast-iron or oven-proof skillet or paella pan and sauté the onion until soft and fragrant.
- Add the garlic and capsicum. Cook until soft, about 5 minutes.
- Mix in tomato paste then tomatoes, smoked paprika and saffron threads (along with the water) and season generously with sea salt and pepper. Cook for a few minutes. Stir in drained rice.
- Add the beans and chickpeas to the simmering vegetable stock to heat through, and then ladle this mixture into your skillet or pan.
- Cook in oven for 20 minutes, or until the rice is tender and the liquid has evaporated.
- Before serving top with artichoke slices and olives.
- Garnish with parsley and serve with lemon wedges on the side.

VARIATION: Instead of brown rice you may prefer to use a traditional short-grain white rice for this dish, like Bomba or Valencia.

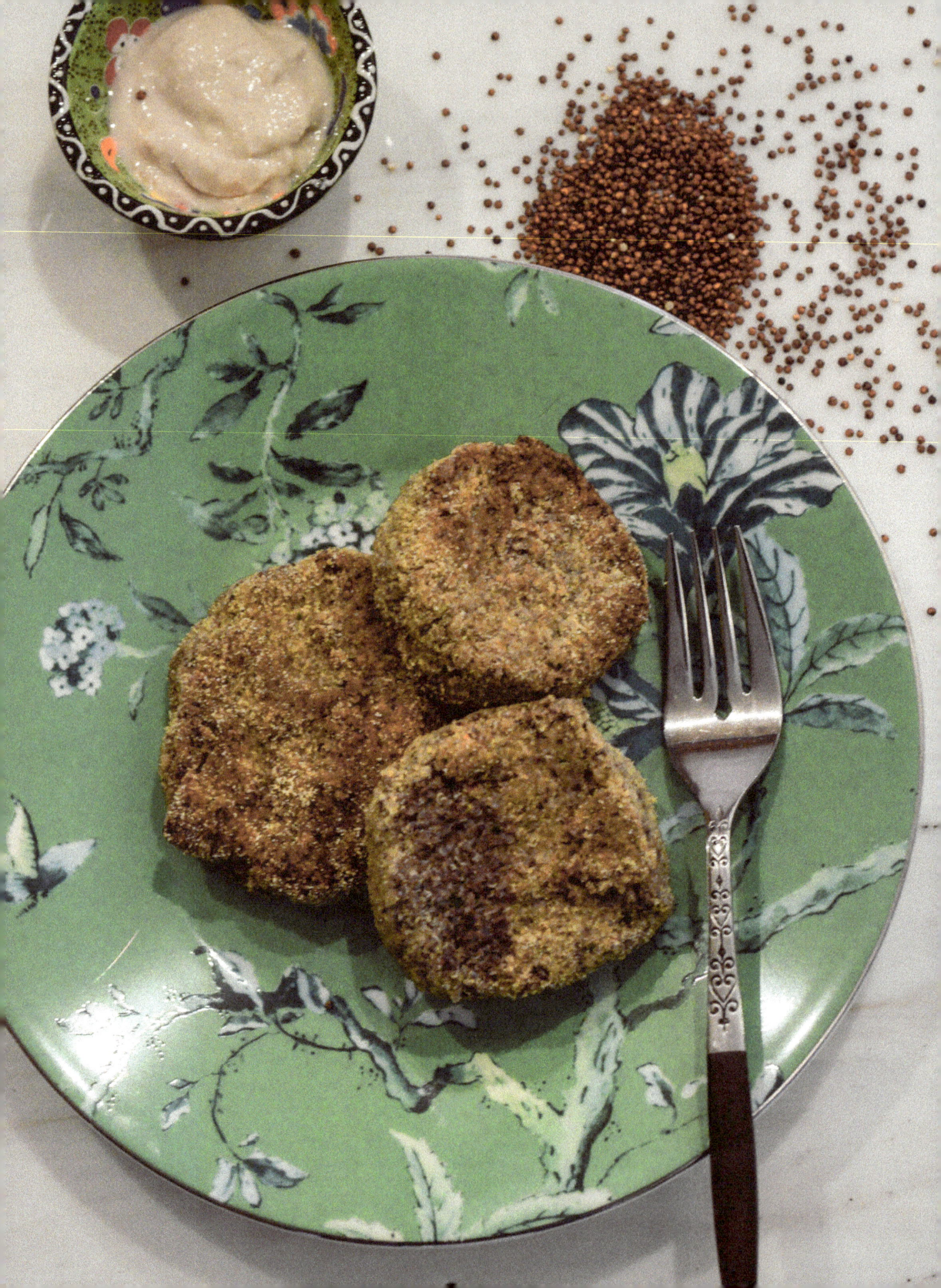

QUINOA BLACK BEAN PATTIES

MAKES 16 X 6 CM PATTIES
LEFTOVERS CAN BE STORED IN AN AIRTIGHT
CONTAINER IN THE REFRIGERATOR FOR UP TO 3 DAYS

4 cups	Cooked quinoa (see tip below)
400 g	Black beans, cooked or tinned, drained
½ cup	Red onion, grated, squeezed dry
1 cup	Coriander, fresh, chopped
1 tbsp	Extra virgin olive oil
2 cloves	Garlic, minced
1 small	Chilli, seeded, finely chopped
1 tsp	Sea salt, to taste
1 tsp	Cumin, ground
1 tsp	Black pepper, ground
2 tbsp	Dulse flakes
⅓ cup	Cornmeal or polenta

- Place cooked quinoa in a food processor with beans, onion, coriander, olive oil, garlic, chilli, sea salt, cumin, pepper and dulse flakes. Puree until well mixed.
- Form into 2 cm–thick patties.
- Place cornmeal or polenta in a shallow bowl and dip patties, coating thoroughly on both sides.
- In a frypan heat a little olive oil then fry patties in batches for about 6 minutes on both sides or until browned.
- Serve with any Dip : Dress : Spread : Top recipe. Miso pesto is a favourite.

Store your cornmeal and polenta in an airtight container in a cool, dry place. I store mine in the refrigerator.

Note: if you prefer, you can use extra virgin coconut oil instead of olive oil

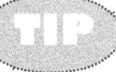

COOKING QUINOA

Wash and drain 1 cup of quinoa very well.

Place in saucepan with 1 ½ cups water and bring to a boil.

Then cover and simmer for 10 minutes until cooked (don't stir).

Remove from heat and leave to steam with lid on for 5 minutes more.

1 cup of dry quinoa = 4 cups cooked grain.

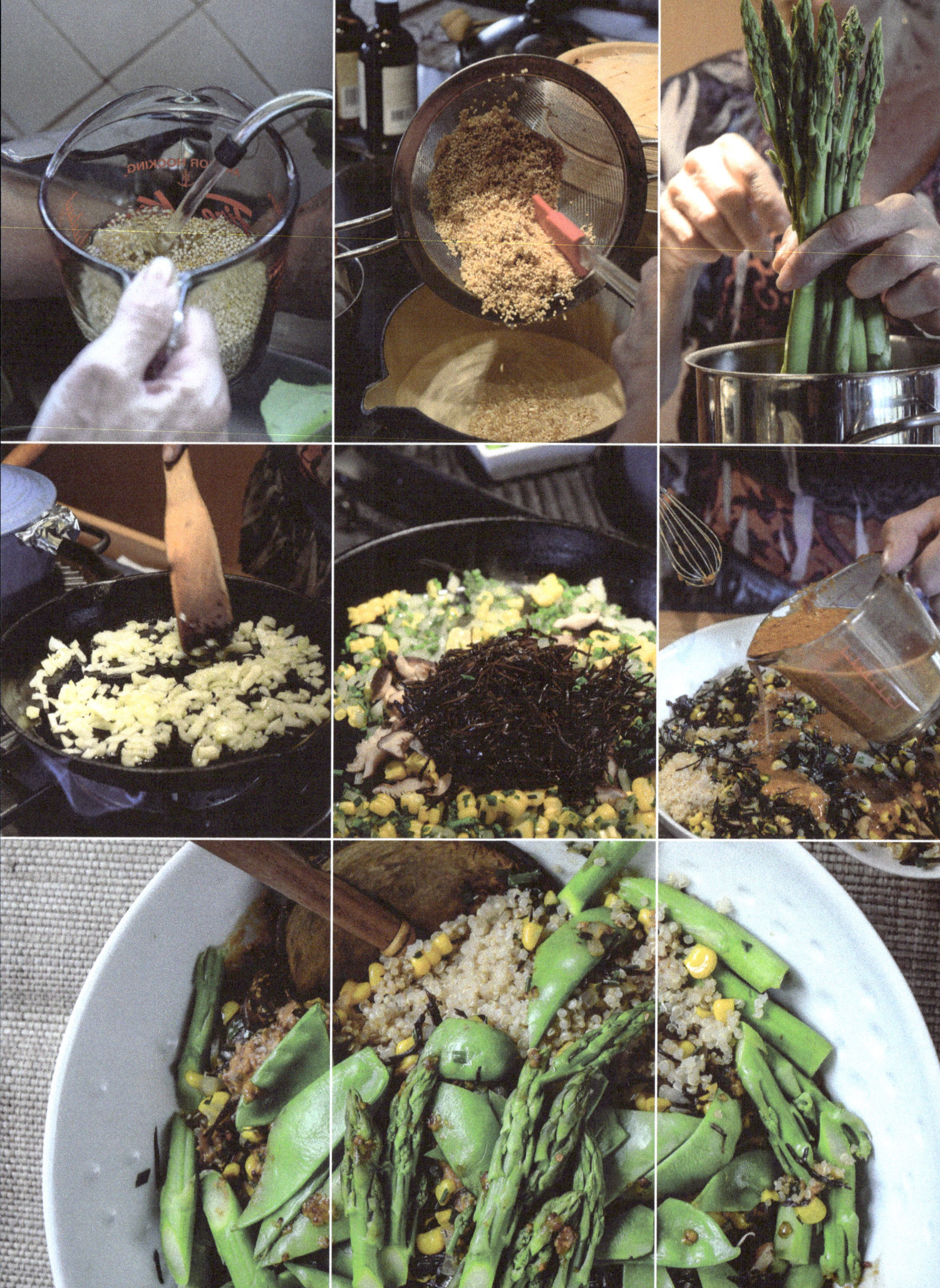

QUINOA CORN ARAME SALAD
With Miso Mustard

SERVES 4
KEEPS REFRIGERATED. BEST USED WITHIN 3 DAYS

5	Shiitake mushrooms, dried
Handful	Arame sea vegetable
8	Asparagus (or use more snow peas or string beans instead)
1 cob	Corn kernels
10	Snow peas or string beans
1 cup	Quinoa
1 ½ cups	Water
Pinch	Sea salt
3 tbsp	Extra virgin olive oil (optional)
1 small	Onion, finely chopped
½–1 bunch	Chives, finely chopped, to taste
3 tbsp	Miso paste (your choice, white for sweetness or dark for saltier flavour)
2–3 tbsp	Mustard, to taste
½–1 cup	Water
½ cup	Walnuts, roasted, chopped

- Soak shiitake mushrooms for at least 30 minutes in 5 cups warm water from the kettle or for even better flavour, soak overnight.
- When mushrooms have softened, discard stems then slice mushrooms caps. Strain shiitake soaking water and keep to use as soup stock.
- Soak arame in enough water to cover for 10 minutes. Strain. Set aside.
- Steam asparagus and corn kernels. Set aside.
- Slice then blanch snow peas or string beans in salted water for 2 minutes. Drain. Set aside.
- Wash quinoa well then place in a saucepan with water and a pinch of sea salt. Bring to boil, cover with lid (don't stir) and reduce heat to simmer for 10 minutes. Remove from heat and leave it to steam with the lid on for 5 minutes. Then place in large serving bowl.
- In a saucepan, fry onions in olive oil or water until translucent.
- Stir in chopped chives, corn kernels, arame and sliced shiitake. Continue frying for 5 minutes then add to cooked quinoa.
- In a small jug, mix miso and mustard with water, then pour about ½ cup of dressing (or more as required) into quinoa mix. (Pour extra dressing into a glass jar and refrigerate for later use.)
- Add snow peas or string beans and asparagus (or more peas or beans).
- Top with chopped roasted walnuts and serve.

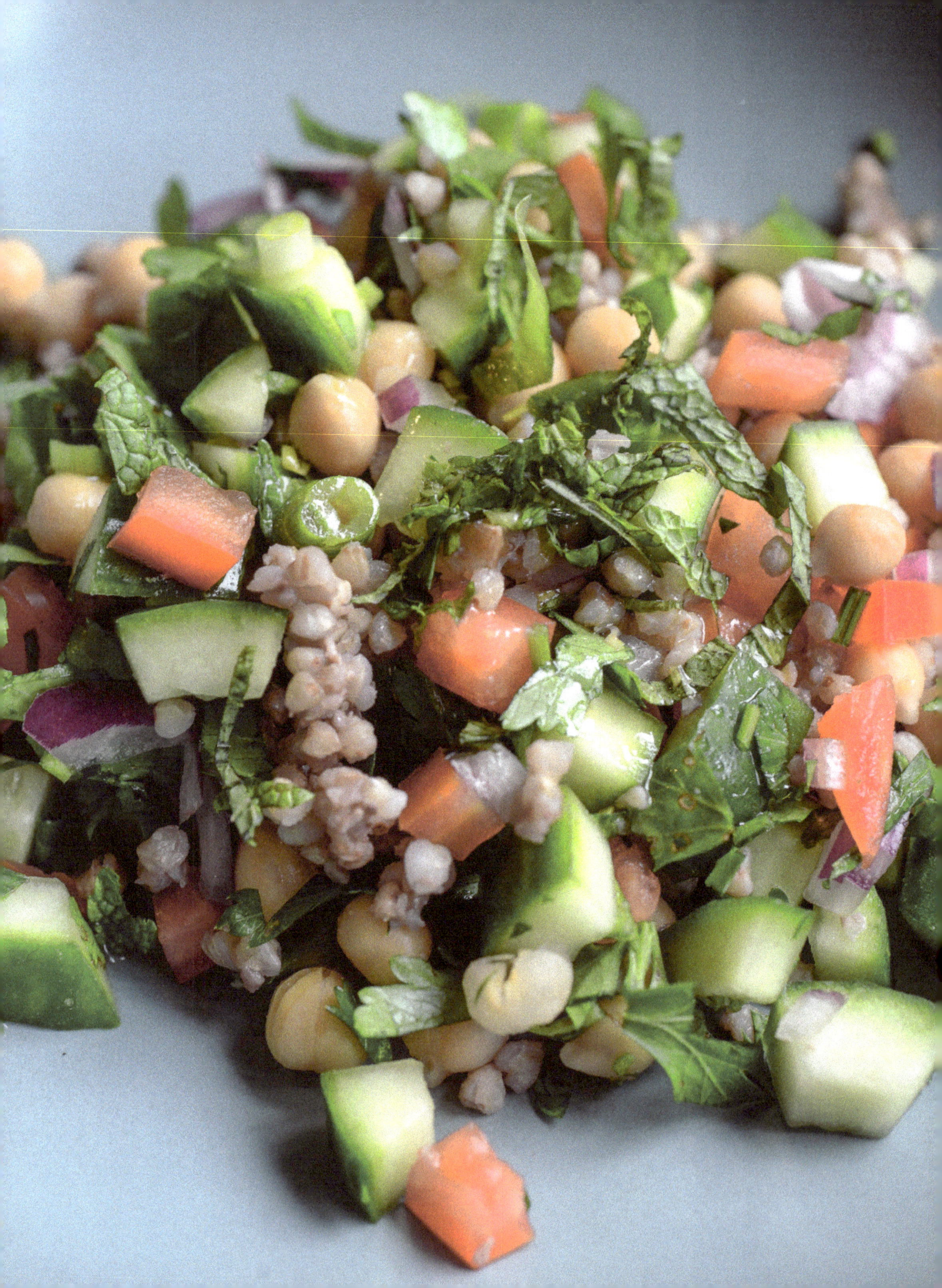

BUCKWHEAT CHICKPEA TABBOULEH

SERVES 4–6
KEEPS FOR 3 DAYS WITHOUT THE DRESSING
(ONLY ADD WHEN SERVING)

1 cup	Buckwheat groats, washed and drained
2 cups	Water
400 g	Chickpeas, cooked or tinned
2 cups	Tomatoes, seeded, cut into small cubes
2 cups	Lebanese cucumber, seeded, quartered and sliced
1 cup	Parsley, fresh, chopped
1 cup	Red onion, finely chopped
¼ cup	Spring onion, finely chopped
½ cup	Mint, fresh, finely chopped

DRESSING

¼ cup	Extra virgin olive oil
3 tbsp	Fresh lemon juice
3 tsp	Plum vinegar (Ume Su)
2 medium	Garlic cloves, minced

- Bring 2 cups water to boil in a medium heavy-based saucepan. Add buckwheat groats then cover, reduce heat to low and simmer for 20 minutes. (Don't stir.)
- Remove from heat and let sit, covered, for 10 minutes. Then remove from saucepan, place in a mixing bowl and fluff to cool.
- When the buckwheat is room temperature, add tomatoes, cucumber, parsley, red onion, spring onion and mint.
- Mix oil, lemon juice, plum vinegar and garlic to make a dressing.
- Pour dressing onto buckwheat salad, add drained cooked chickpeas and mix through.
- Serve at room temperature.

As a holistic health practitioner (Osteopath and have diplomas in both Naturopathy and Acupuncture) I have always been driven by the desire to heal the whole. Twenty years ago was my first class with Sandra and she opened up a whole new world of possibilities in my cooking that I have continued to implement in my own way since. Her classes were like a fresh new world to me. Plant-based whole foods and Japanese-style cooking use many unusual ingredients that are a rich source of minerals that have helped improve my diet. Ingredients like mirin and tamari are so easy to include in vegie dishes and they revolutionise the taste of a broth.

Dr Mike Rowan, Melbourne

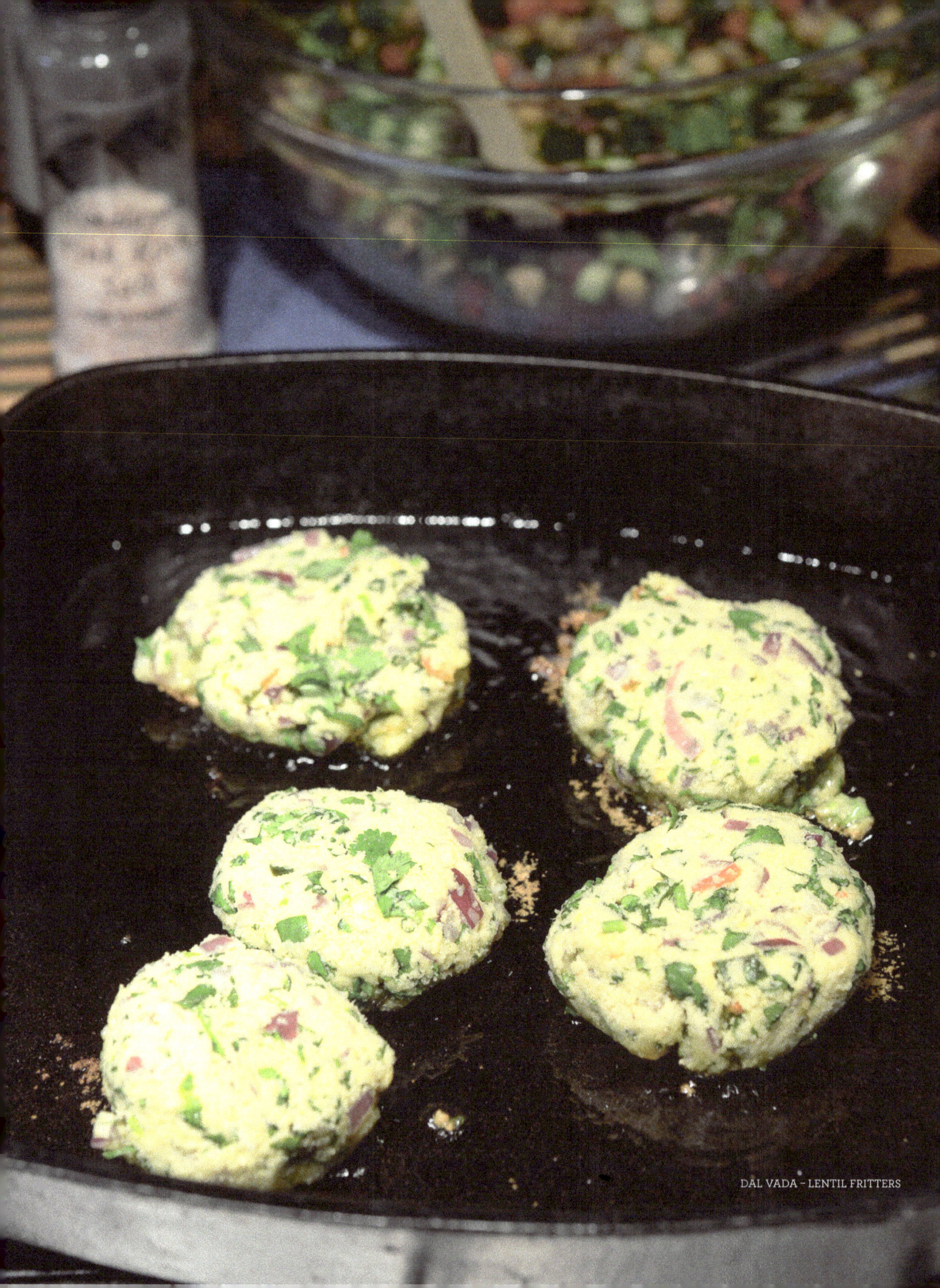

DĀL VADA – LENTIL FRITTERS

Nutritious Legumes

Kidney Bean Salad 97

Moroccan Chickpea Carrot Tagine 98

Adzuki Bean Vegetable Stew 101

Chickpea Polenta 102

Thai Tofu Vegetable Patties.. 103

Thai Tofu Sweet Potato Curry.. 105

Tofu Scramble – San Choy Bau.. 105

Dal Vada – Lentil Fritters 107

Slow Cooked Curried Dahl 107

Tempeh And Tofu Mustard... 109

Black Bean Aztec Salad.. 109

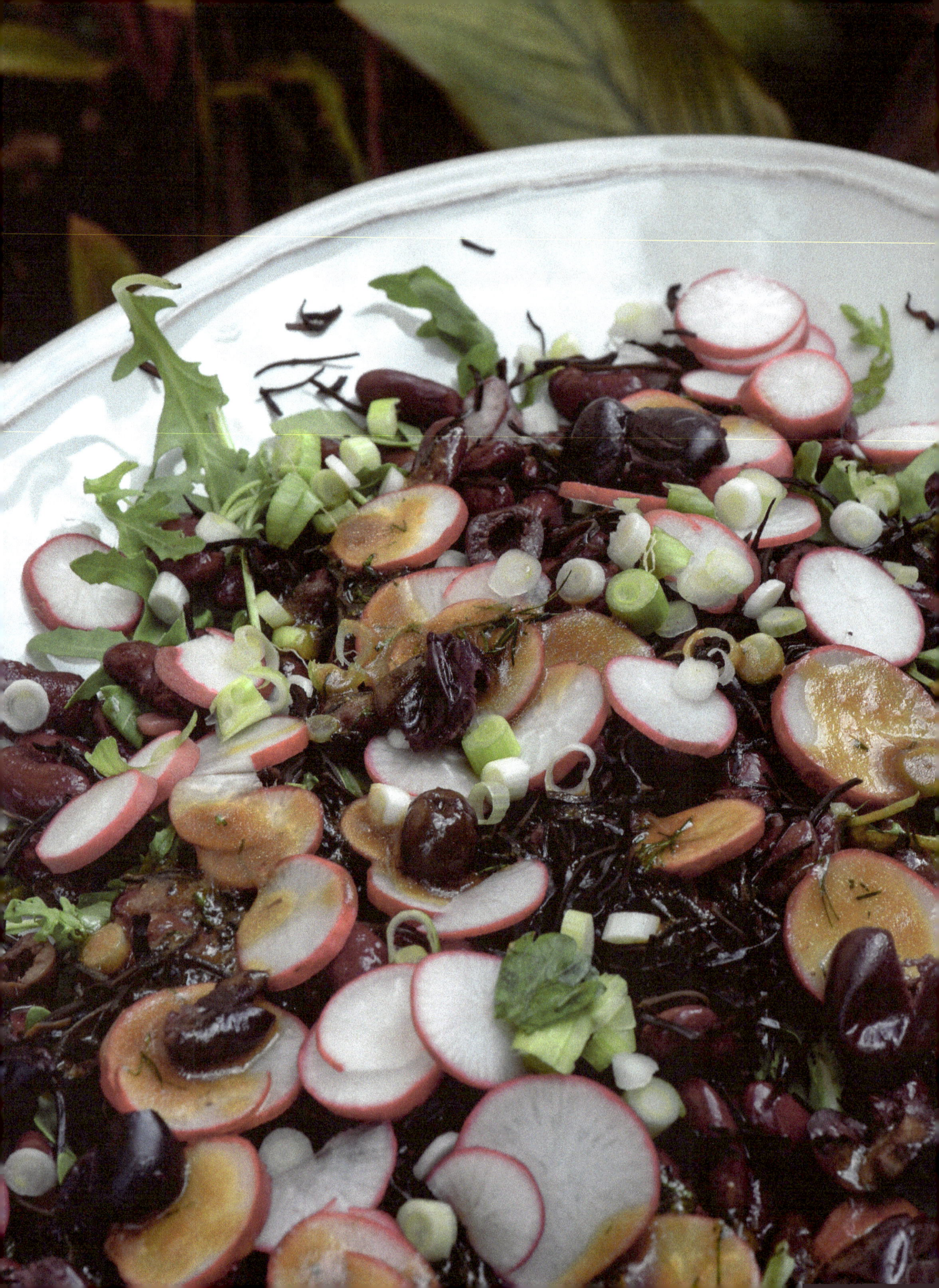

TIP: BEAN COOKING SECRETS (FROM ONE OF MY MENTORS)

Organic beans are preferred. Rinse dried beans and pick out any loose stones. Place beans in a large bowl, cover with hot water and let them soak. Soaking time varies depending on the bean variety and freshness, and can range from 2 to 24 hours. Black turtle, borlotti, broad, cannelini (great northern), chickpeas, kidney, lima, navy and pinto are best soaked overnight. Before cooking discard soaking water. Rinse beans again.

Layer 10 cm strip of kombu sea vegetable, or if you can't find kombu, use kelp or wakame sea vegetable, on the bottom of a heavy based cooking pot. Place soaked, strained beans and fresh cold water into the pot and bring to a boil, then cover and reduce heat to simmer until tender.

Boiling toughens beans, so simmer them slowly. (Or cook in a pressure cooker, a convenient and healthy way to feed your family while still preserving the nutrients in your food). At the beginning of cooking, skim off and discard any foam that rises to the top of the pot.

Add seasonings to aid digestibility. The herbs asafoetida, cumin, epazote, fennel and ginger enhance digestion of beans. I also add a 10 cm strip of kombu per cup of dry beans; a natural source of glutamic acid, kombu tenderises, enhances flavour and adds invaluable vitamins and minerals. It also helps to reduce the gas-producing properties of beans. After an hour or so of cooking beans, the kombu will disintegrate when stirred. (Any stray pieces should be tender enough to eat, or you can remove them.)

Cook beans until softened and then add ½ teaspoon sea salt per cup of dry beans before serving.

KIDNEY BEAN SALAD

SERVES 4-6
KEEPS REFRIGERATED FOR 3 DAYS

⅓ cup	Arame sea vegetable
400 g	Kidney beans, cooked or tinned, drained
4	Spring onions, finely chopped
6	Red radishes, sliced into thin discs
½ cup	Olives, pitted
3–4 cups	Watercress or rocket, chopped
1 quantity	Miso dill dressing (see recipe p.42)

- Soak arame in boiled hot water for 10 minutes, then drain.
- In a large salad bowl, add cooked beans, finely chopped spring onions, sliced radish, pitted olives, chopped watercress or rocket and softened arame.
- Toss through miso dill dressing and serve.

MOROCCAN CHICKPEA CARROT TAGINE

SERVES 3–4

1	Onion, chopped
3–4	Garlic cloves, minced, to taste
3 tbsp	Extra virgin olive oil
2 tsp	Ginger, grated
1 tsp	Turmeric, grated
½ tsp	Black pepper, ground
½–1 tsp	Cayenne pepper, to taste
1 tsp	Ras el hanout spice mix
½ cup	Coriander or parsley, fresh, chopped
4 medium	Carrots, cut into 3 cm lengths
1 cup	Water or vegetable stock (see recipe)
400 g	Chickpeas, cooked or tinned, drained
1 tbsp	Honey or other liquid sweetener
1–2 tsp	Sea salt, to taste
Garnish	Coriander or parsley
Garnish	Almonds, chopped

- In the base of a tagine or in a large pot with a lid, sauté onions and garlic in oil over low heat for 5 minutes.
- Add spices, fresh coriander or parsley, carrots and water or stock.
- Cover and simmer over low heat until the carrots are cooked to desired tenderness. (In a large pot this may take up to 20 minutes; in a tagine, a bit longer.)
- When the carrots are cooked, stir in the sweetener and chickpeas.
- Continue simmering until the chickpeas are heated through.
- Adjust seasoning to your taste, add garnish and serve with brown rice or hulled millet (see recipes).

I first met Sandy through a mutual friend in about 2002. I enrolled in Sandy's group cooking class that was given in her home. I loved the intimate, warm atmosphere and setting. I especially enjoyed the delicious food and was introduced to a lot of foods and information I had never heard of before. Sandy has an engaging personality and everything was fun. The thing I remember most is seeing miso paste for the first time and making real miso soup. I have enjoyed making it for myself and friends over the years. I also became very knowledgeable about good quality oils and how and when to use them.

Later I did other group classes with Sandy including traditional Japanese cooking classes, private classes with my staff and bought her inspiring cooking video (made in 1999) to make lots of dishes from that too. When my daughter had her 13th birthday (12 years ago) Sandy gave a special Japanese cooking demonstration for her and about 15 of her friends in my home. All the kids were involved in making a sushi roll and they loved it. Thanks Sandy for all the wonderful lessons and your sharing of delicious wholesome food and nutritional information with me.

Roslyn Eldar, Company Director, Melbourne

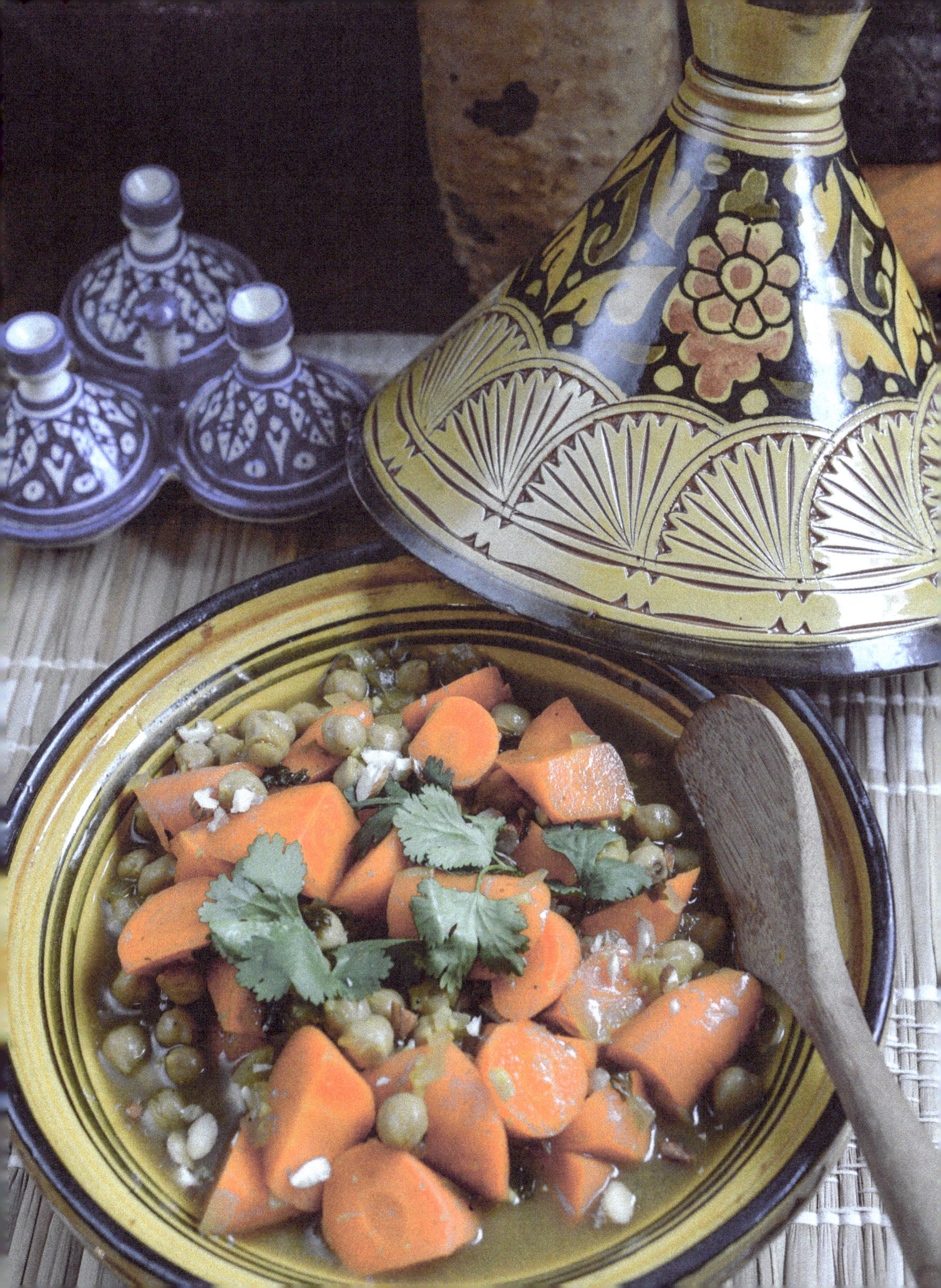

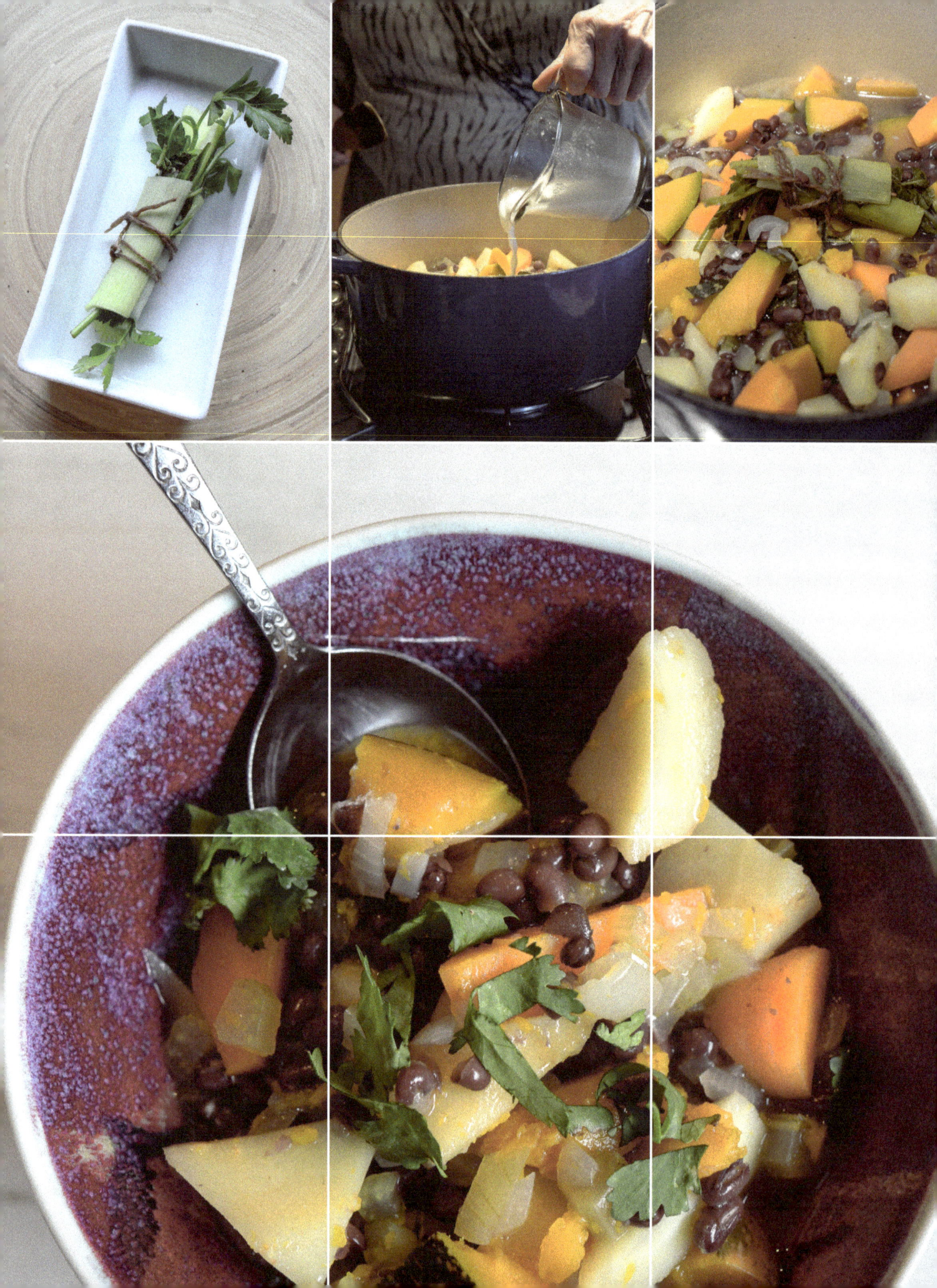

ADZUKI BEAN VEGETABLE STEW

SERVES 4

1 clove	Garlic, minced
1 large	Onion, chopped
1 strip	Kombu or wakame sea vegetable, rinsed
1 cup	Adzuki beans, dried, soaked for 3 hours
1	Bouquet garni (see below)
1 large	Carrot, large diced
1 small	Parsnip, large diced
2 cups	Japanese pumpkin, seeded, large diced (keep skin on)
1 cup	Celery, diced
Pinch	Sea salt
2 tbsp	Kuzu starch, dissolved in ¼ cup of cold water

BOUQUET GARNI

2	Bay leaves
3 sprigs	Thyme or basil
4 large	Parsley sprigs (including stalks)
10 cm	Celery, stalk with leaves
2 x 10 cm	Leek, green part

- Rinse soaked adzuki beans and pick over to ensure no rocks are present.
- Fry onions and garlic in a little water in a large saucepan until golden brown, add kombu or wakame and adzuki beans. Cover with water.
- Bring to the boil and simmer for 30 minutes, adding a little more water occasionally to keep beans covered.
- Add the vegetables and bouquet garni to the beans as well as enough water to fill ⅓ of the saucepan. Let simmer for another 30 minutes.
- Remove bouquet garni, add sea salt, then simmer for an additional 10 minutes.
- Add dissolved kuzu to pot and stir until it becomes transparent.
- Adjust seasoning to your taste and serve.

BOUQUET GARNI

- Place bay leaves, thyme or basil, parsley and celery on one piece of green leek. Cover with the remaining piece of green leek.
- Tie securely with fine string, leaving a length of string attached so that the bouquet garni can be easily retrieved.

I had the pleasure of being Sandy's assistant, so I attended many classes and learnt so so much. One of my favourite recipes is the kidney bean/arame/dill salad with miso dressing. I have made this dish so many times, adding different ingredients at different times, seeds, leafy greens... I've taken it dinner parties and picnics and it always gets a 'wow delicious!!' Plus of course the classic adzuki and pumpkin dish that could heal the world! I really appreciate learning the integrating of new ingredients and methods into my daily cooking... arame, shiitake mushrooms, miso dressings, soaking brown rice, kombu in soups and stews, umeboshi in dressings, using these Japanese ingredients in a fusion way.

I have discovered that this layered, nutritious, delicious way of cooking can be so easy, being creative and flexible in the kitchen. Sandy's style is specific and committed but also free flexible and fun - a winning combination.

Mia Rappel, MIAMIA, Design, Installation, Visual Arts, Events, Melbourne

CHICKPEA POLENTA

SERVES 4

2 cups	Water
1 tsp	Sea salt
¼ tsp	Black pepper, ground
¼ tsp	Garlic powder or onion powder
¼ tsp	Cumin
¼ cup	Extra virgin olive oil
120 g	Besan (chickpea) flour
2 tbsp	Parsley or basil, fresh, chopped
To fry	Extra virgin olive oil

- Pour water, sea salt, pepper, garlic or onion powder, cumin and oil into a heavy-based saucepan over medium heat and whisk in besan flour until smooth.
- Keep cooking and stirring, making sure to scrape the bottom and sides of pan, until mixture is stiff and starts to pull away from the sides as you stir. This takes about 10 minutes.
- Place the batter into an oiled glass or sealed ceramic heatproof dish (about 20 x 15 cm) and quickly spread it with a spatula before it cools and sets. (A handy tip is to dip your spatula in cold water to help you spread.)
- Allow to cool until completely firm, then cut into pieces.
- Pour enough olive oil into a heavy-based skillet to cover the bottom with ½ cm of oil and heat. Fry pieces of polenta for about 3 minutes on each side until golden and crisp.
- Serve warm with sweet and sour arame or tofu beetroot dip.

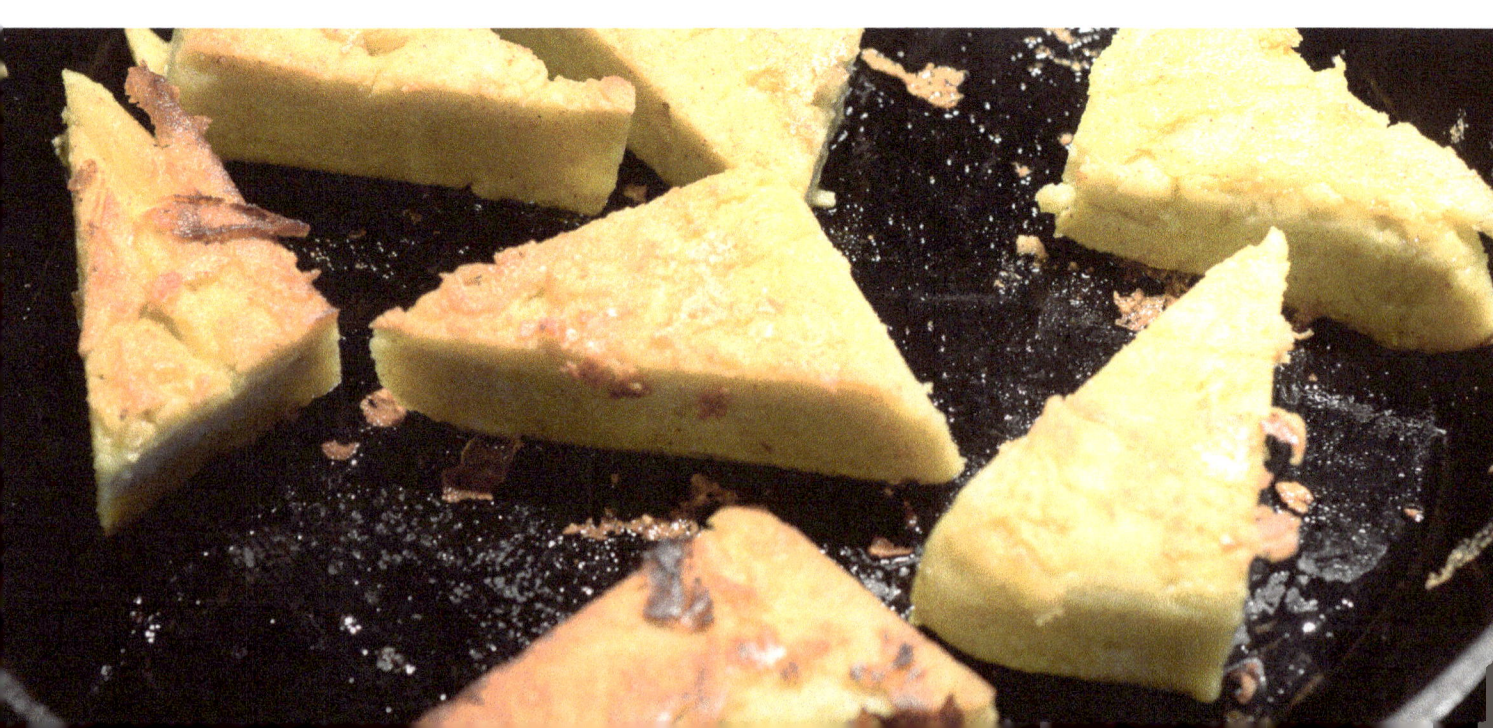

THAI TOFU VEGETABLE PATTIES

MAKES 12–15 4 CM PATTIES
LEFTOVERS CAN BE STORED IN AN AIRTIGHT CONTAINER IN THE REFRIGERATOR FOR UP TO 3 DAYS

250 g	Tofu, firm
4	Shiitake mushrooms, dried
15 g	Arame sea vegetable
150 g	Sweet potato, peeled or scrubbed with skin
1 medium	Onion, chopped
4	Baby corn, chopped
1 small	Carrot, grated
1 tsp	Black pepper, ground
½ tsp	Sea salt
4 cloves	Garlic, halved
15 g	Coriander, fresh
5 cm	Lemongrass, finely sliced
50 ml	Water
4 tbsp	Brown rice flour
For frying	Coconut oil
1 quantity	Almond satay sauce

I prefer the flavour of dried Japanese shiitake mushrooms – see glossary.

- Place tofu in bowl, cover with boiled hot water and soak for 5 minutes. Drain.
- Soak shiitake mushrooms for at least 30 minutes in 5 cups warm water from the kettle or for even better flavour, soak overnight. Discard stems and slice shiitake caps.
- Soak arame for 10 minutes, drain and chop
- Steam sweet potato then mash. (A bamboo steamer is best.)
- Place vegetables, including sweet potato and mushrooms, soaked arame, drained tofu, pepper, sea salt, garlic, coriander and lemongrass in a food processor. Blend into paste.
- Put the paste into a saucepan and cook over a gentle heat for 3 minutes, stirring constantly.
- Mix water and rice flour together and add a little of it to the paste. Continue to stir over gentle heat and add more rice flour and water if needed. Remove from heat and leave to cool.
- Form mixture into small 4 cm patties and chill in refrigerator for 15 minutes.
- Heat oil in wok. Fry patties for 2 to 3 minutes until golden brown. Remove and drain.
- If you prefer to bake, as I did for the photo, then place patties in a pre-heated 200°C oven (my oven is electric) for about 10 minutes, or until golden brown.
- Serve with almond satay sauce (see recipe p.43).

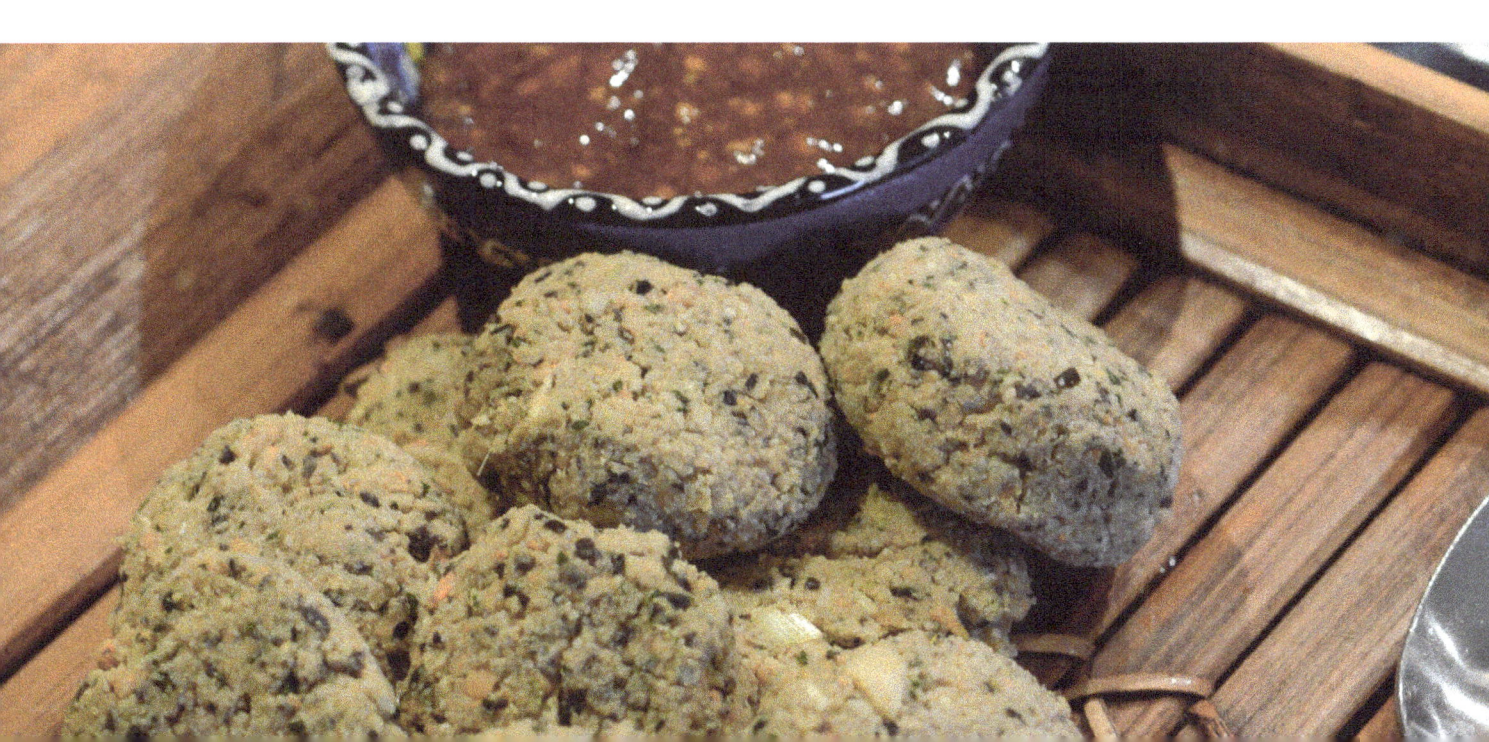

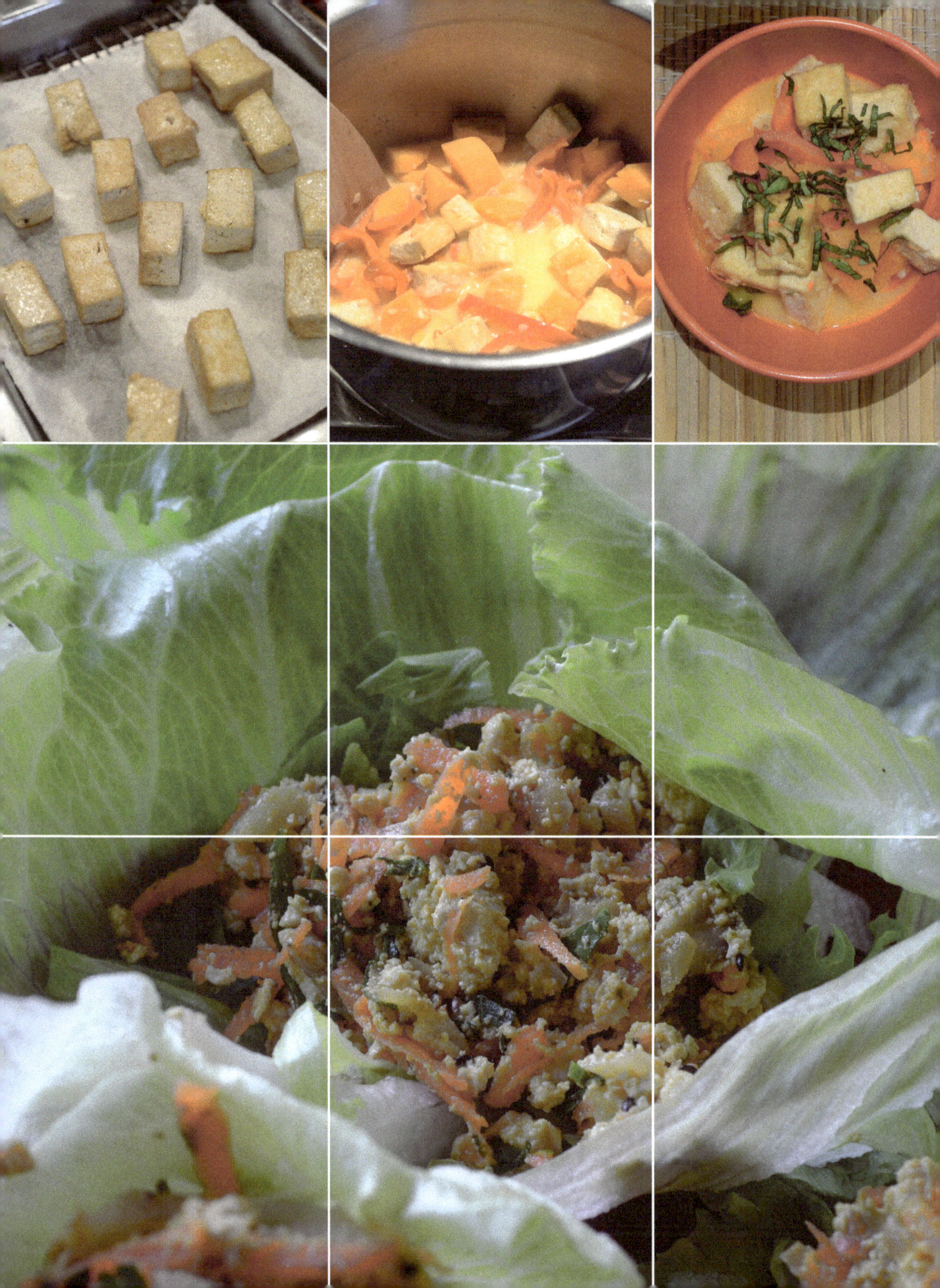

THAI TOFU SWEET POTATO CURRY

SERVES 4

500 g	Tofu, firm
4 tsp	Coconut oil
1 tbsp	Ginger, fresh, grated
3	Garlic cloves, minced
½ cup	Coconut milk
¾ cup	Water
2 tsp	Red curry paste (see recipe p.43)
To taste	Sea salt
500 g	Sweet potato, peeled, cut into 3 cm cubes
1 medium	Red capsicum, seeded, chopped
10 large	Thai basil leaves, cut into thin strips

- Place tofu in bowl, cover with boiled hot water and soak for 5 minutes. Drain.
- Slice tofu into 3 cm slabs and wrap in a clean cotton cloth. Place under a light chopping board for 5 minutes to help drain excess water from tofu. (This prevents oil splattering while frying.) Remove from cloth and cut tofu into 3 cm cubes.
- Heat oil in large frypan over medium-high heat. Add tofu cubes, reduce heat to medium, and cook, turning occasionally, until golden brown, about 5 minutes. Remove tofu to a draining tray.
- Add ginger and garlic to empty saucepan and cook until fragrant, about 30 seconds. Add coconut milk, water, red curry paste and sea salt. Bring to a boil, stirring to dissolve curry paste.
- Add sweet potato cubes and chopped capsicum, cover then reduce heat to simmer, stirring once or twice, until vegetables are tender, about 10 minutes.
- Add tofu to this mix and simmer, uncovered, until sauce thickens slightly, about 2 minutes.
- Adjust seasonings and garnish with Thai basil.
- Serve with cooked brown rice or noodles.

TOFU SCRAMBLE – SAN CHOY BAU

SERVES 4–6

4	Shiitake mushrooms, dried or fresh
250 g	Tofu
½ tsp	Turmeric, ground
1 tbsp	Tamari or shoyu OR 2 tbsp white miso paste (Shiro – my choice for this recipe)
⅓ cup	Shiitake soaking water or water, as required
1 tbsp	Toasted sesame oil
¼ cup	Fennel, diced OR 3 tbsp chives, chopped
1 tbsp	Dulse flakes OR sea vegetable seasoning (I use Furikake seasoning from Spiral Foods)
1 small	Carrot, shredded
½ cup	Parsley, chopped
3 tbsp	Chives (optional)
For serving	Iceberg lettuce leaves

- If using dried shiitake: Soak shiitake mushrooms for at least 30 minutes in 5 cups warm water from the kettle (see tip, p55) or for even better flavour, soak overnight. Strain soaking water and keep. Discard stems and slice shiitake caps.
- If using fresh shiitake, slice.
- Mash tofu, turmeric, tamari or shoyu or miso paste together. Add shiitake soaking water or water if needed to blend.
- Heat oil in a small wok. If using diced fennel, add here. If using fresh mushrooms, add and sauté.
- Add tofu puree and flakes or seasoning. If using dried shiitake, then add here. Add a little more liquid for a smoother texture.
- Add shredded carrots and chopped parsley.
- Cook uncovered for 10 minutes, stirring occasionally.
- If using chives, add near end of cooking.
- Serve in lettuce leaves.

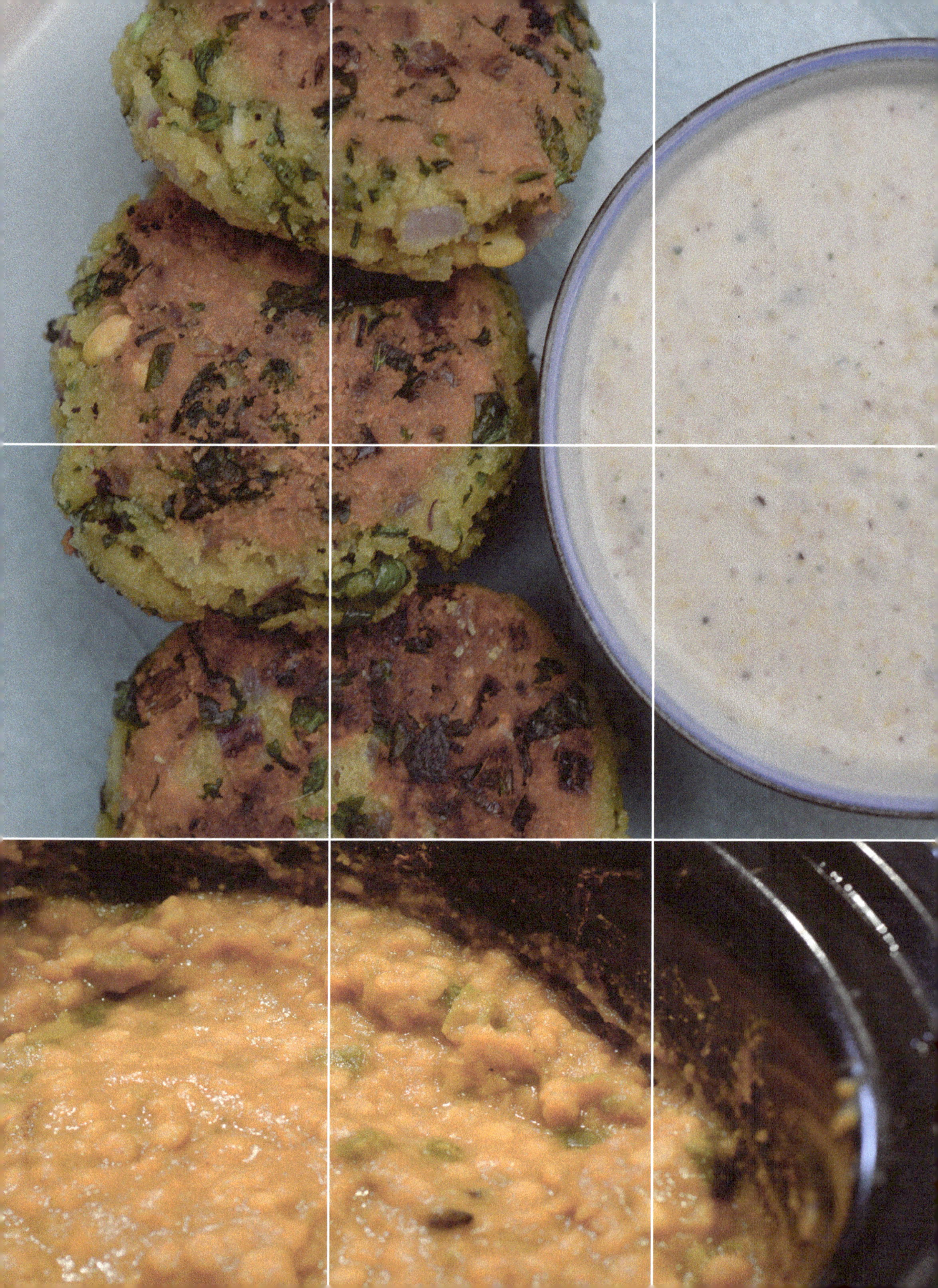

This recipe inspired by friend and Master Chef Jitendra Bhatia.

DAL VADA – LENTIL FRITTERS

MAKES 6 LARGE OR 10 SMALL CRUNCHY FRITTERS

200 g	Chana dal
Pinch	Sea salt
1	Onion, finely chopped (or use fennel)
1	Green chilli, finely chopped (optional)
¼ bunch	Coriander, finely chopped
To taste	Ginger, grated
1–2 cloves	Garlic, minced, to taste
For frying	Coconut or sesame oil

- Wash chana dal and soak overnight.
- Before using, rinse and drain chana dal. Then, using a food processor or mortar and pestle, grind dal with a pinch of salt to a coarse or smooth texture, as you prefer.
- Add finely chopped vegetables, ginger and garlic to taste. Mix well, adding more water if required.
- Shape mixture into patties.
- Heat oil in frypan and cook patties on each side for a couple of minutes until browned and crispy.
- Serve with coconut chutney (see recipe p.127) or any sauce (see Dip : Dress : Spread : Top section).

SLOW COOKED CURRIED DAHL
With Sweet Potato

SERVES 4-8

300 g	Split peas, dried (yellow, red or green – it's up to you)
1 medium	Green capsicum, seeded, diced
2 cups	Sweet potato, peeled and grated
5 cups	Vegetable stock
1	Bay leaf
1–2	*Chipotle chillies in adobo, sliced OR 1–2 tsp smoked paprika
1	Star anise
½–1 tsp	Curry powder
1 tbsp	Tamari
½ tsp	Black pepper, ground
2–3 cloves	Garlic, minced, to taste

- Place ingredients in a slow cooker and cook at a low setting for 8 hours, then add a cup of water and turn heat to high setting for about another hour. Cook until peas begin to fall apart.
- Adjust seasonings as required then serve.

Chipotle in adobo is a rich, smoky, spicy Mexican sauce (adobo) made of smoke-dried, ripe jalapeno chillies (chipotle). It's really hot and has a smoky flavour.

Delicious with homemade vegetable stock. Recipe for stock p.16.

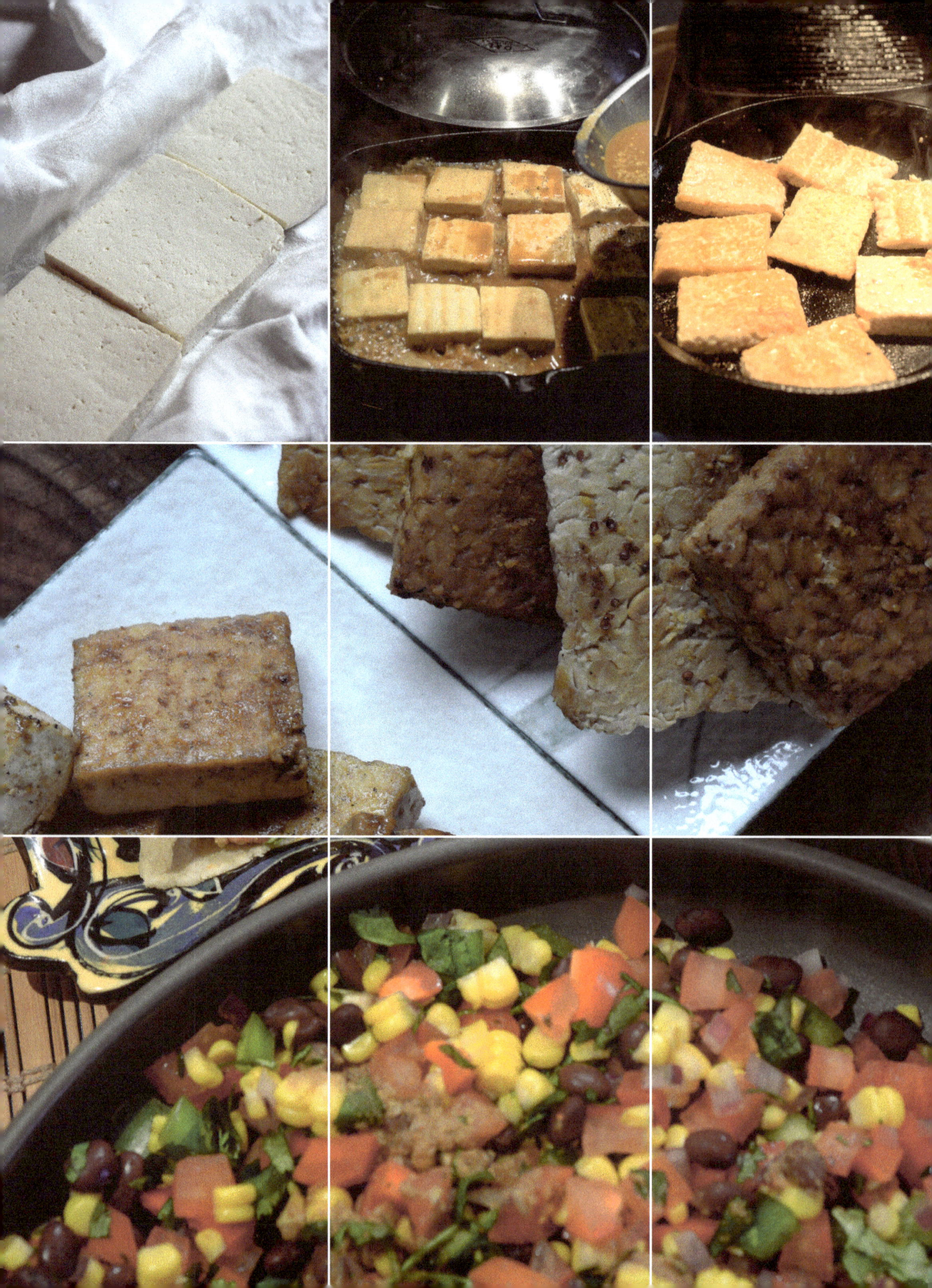

TEMPEH AND TOFU MUSTARD

SERVES 4
KEEPS REFRIGERATED FOR 3 DAYS

250–300 g	Tempeh and/or tofu
1 tbsp	Coconut, sesame or extra virgin olive oil
2 tbsp	Mustard
2 tsp	Tamari
1 cup	Water
½ cup	Fresh basil leaves, chopped

- If using tempeh: Slice tempeh in half so it becomes half as thick, then cut into quarters.
- If using tofu: Wrap 2 cm slabs of tofu in a clean cotton cloth and place under a light chopping board for 5 minutes to help drain excess water from tofu. Remove from cloth then cut into 6 cm squares.
- Heat oil in a frypan, add tempeh and/or tofu and brown on each side.
- In a separate bowl, whisk together mustard, tamari and water.
- Pour mustard mixture over the browned tempeh and/or tofu, cover pan with lid, reduce heat to low and simmer for about 10 minutes or until most of the liquid has evaporated.
- Cut tempeh and or tofu into smaller pieces, if desired, and serve hot or cool and garnished with basil.

BLACK BEAN AZTEC SALAD

SERVES 4–6
YOU CAN MAKE THIS IN ADVANCE AS IT KEEPS WELL FOR SEVERAL DAYS

400 g	Black beans, cooked, rinsed and drained
½ cup	Red onion, finely chopped
1 medium	Green capsicum, seeded, diced
1 medium	Red or yellow capsicum, seeded, diced
2 cups	Corn kernels, fresh, cooked
2 large	Tomatoes, diced (you can seed tomatoes if you prefer)
¾ cup	Coriander, fresh, chopped (or parsley)
3 tbsp	Brown rice vinegar
2 tbsp	Apple cider vinegar
1	Lemon or lime, juiced
2 cloves	Garlic, pressed or finely minced
2 tsp	Cumin, ground
1 tsp	Coriander, ground
½ tsp	Chilli flakes or a pinch of cayenne
1	*Chipotle chilli in adobo sauce, diced or any salsa (I like to use Salsa de Habanero by Ranchero with a little added smoked paprika)

- In a large bowl, combine beans, onion, capsicums, corn, tomatoes and coriander.
- In a small bowl, whisk together vinegars, lemon or lime juice, garlic, ground cumin, ground coriander, chilli flakes or cayenne, and chipotle or salsa.
- Pour over salad and toss gently to mix.
- Serve with corn tortillas (see recipe p.128).

Chipotle in adobo is a rich, smoky, spicy Mexican sauce (adobo) made of smoke-dried, ripe jalapeno chillies (chipotle). It's really hot and has a smoky flavour.

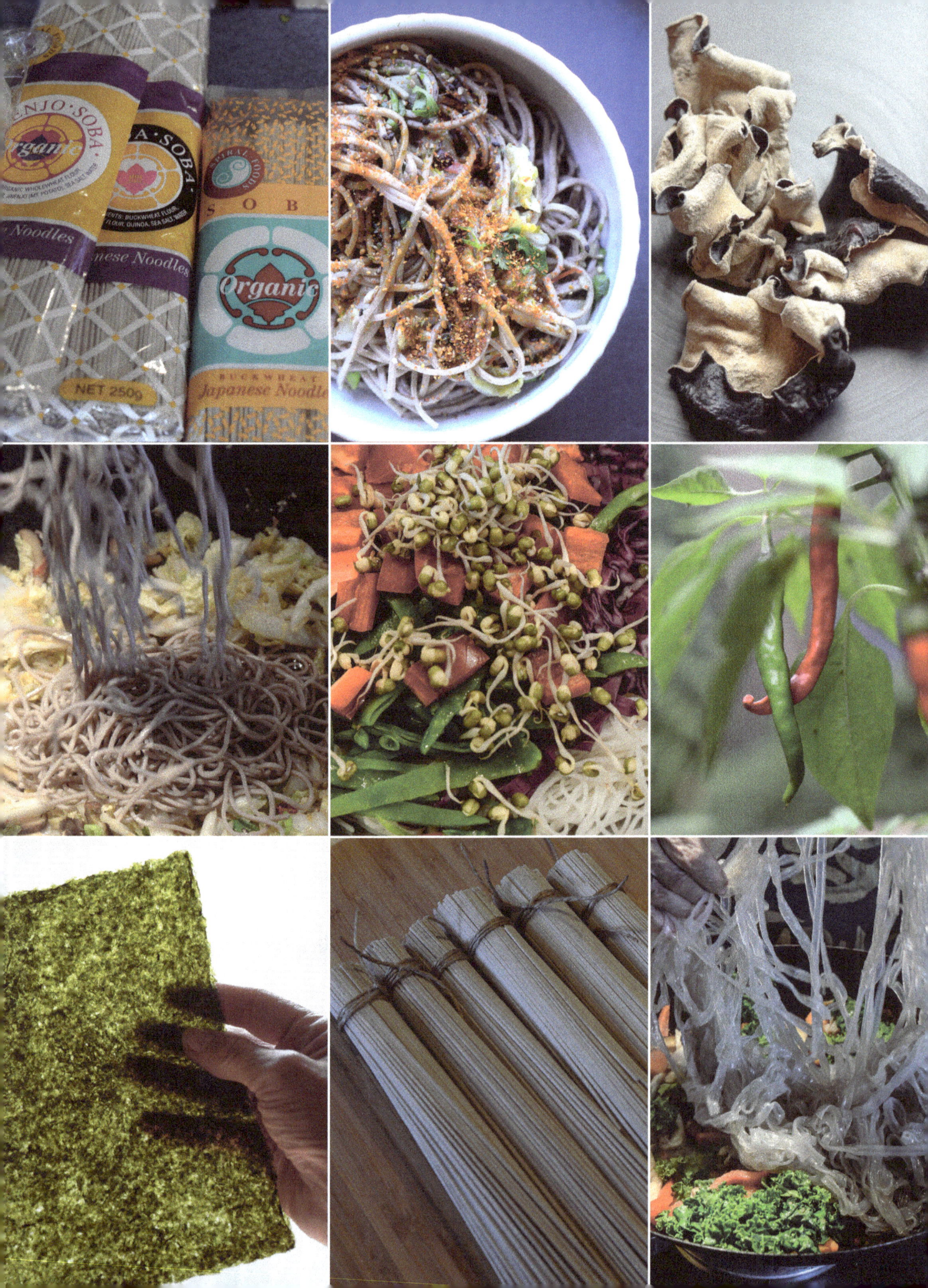

Salubrious Noodles

Noodle Nori Rolls	113
Soba Noodle Stir Fry	115
Sweet Potato Noodle Stir Fry	117
Rice Or Bean Noodle Salad	119
Chiang Mai Vegetable Noodle	121

I was personally excited when Sandra told me the time had come for the often spoken about collective stories to be published. I've been happy to be associated with Sandra and we go back a long way – it's fantastic that her passion for food has never faded. Sandra's enthusiasm is infectious and it comes out with all projects that she involves herself in.

Sandra has had a rich and successful career within the wholefoods industry. She has run her own wholefoods café/store, the famous Japanese cooking school and her ever successful intimate wholefood cooking circle and mixed this with lectures, studying, consultations and seminars to just offering friendly advice to those she meets on food and diet. All these ingredients make the perfect recipe for My Wholefood Community Cookbook. A must for those who feel that WHOLESOME FOOD MATTERS!

James Wilson, Spiral Foods, Melbourne

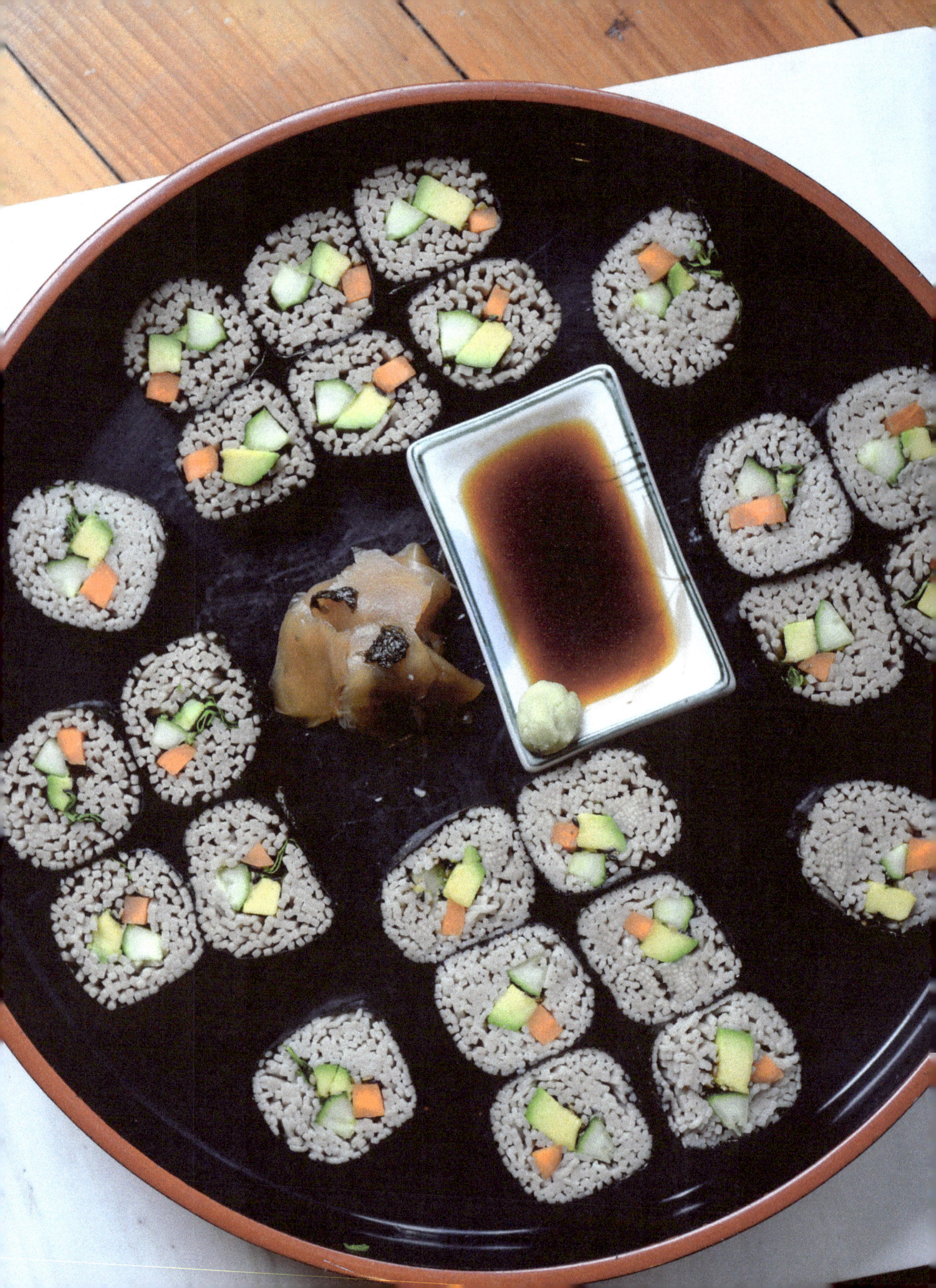

Get your bamboo sushi mat ready to roll!

NOODLE NORI ROLLS

MAKES ABOUT 18 SMALL NORI ROLLS

250 g	Soba or udon noodles (or gluten-free noodles)
3 sheets	Toasted sushi nori
1	Avocado, sliced
1	Continental cucumber, seeded and sliced into long strips
1	Carrot, julienned, parboiled in water with tamari or shoyu
To taste	Pickled ginger
To taste	Toasted sesame seeds
To taste	Fresh mint, coriander, basil or chives
	String (to tie noodle bundles)

DIPPING SAUCE

1 tbsp	Tamari or shoyu
1 tbsp	Water
1 tsp	Mirin
1 tsp	Wasabi paste (I recommend using natural wasabi powder without artificial additives)

Don't overpower delicate flavours of your nori roll with too much soy dipping sauce.

- Divide the uncooked noodles into 3 bundles and tie each bundle firmly with string about 2 cm from one end only. (You can make larger rolls by using more noodles in a bundle.)
- Drop the noodle bundles – string side first – into a large pot of boiling water and cook until just tender. Once ready, drain noodles and plunge into cold water. Drain again.
- Place a sheet of toasted nori, rough side facing you, on a sushi mat.
- Place noodles across bottom ⅓ of nori, leaving at least a 5 cm margin from the bottom of the sheet. Cut off the ends where the noodles are tied and spread the noodles across the nori sheet.
- Place a variety of fillings (i.e. avocado, cucumber, carrot, ginger, seeds and herbs) in the centre of the noodles and press in with your fingers.
- Place thumbs under bamboo mat and fingers on top of fillings and roll the mat over the ingredients, compress ingredients into a square shape.
- Move the mat forward and continue rolling until you reach the end of the nori. Put pressure on the roll from all three sides at all times to ensure it rolls tightly. Make sure you tighten the roll moving from the ends to the centre so as not to squeeze out the roll filling.
- Let the roll rest for a couple of minutes and repeat the process with the remaining noodles.
- Dip the blade of a sharp knife in cold water then slice each roll into 4–6 pieces.
- Mix together all ingredients for the dipping sauce and serve with rolls.

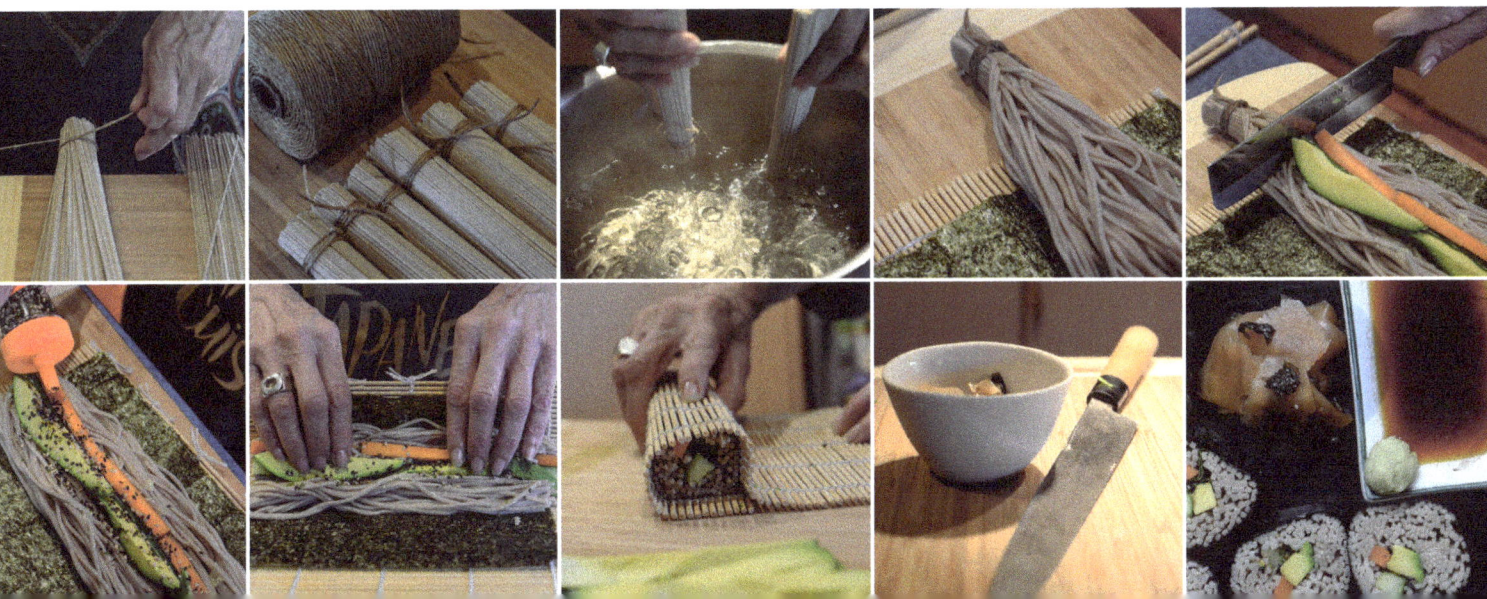

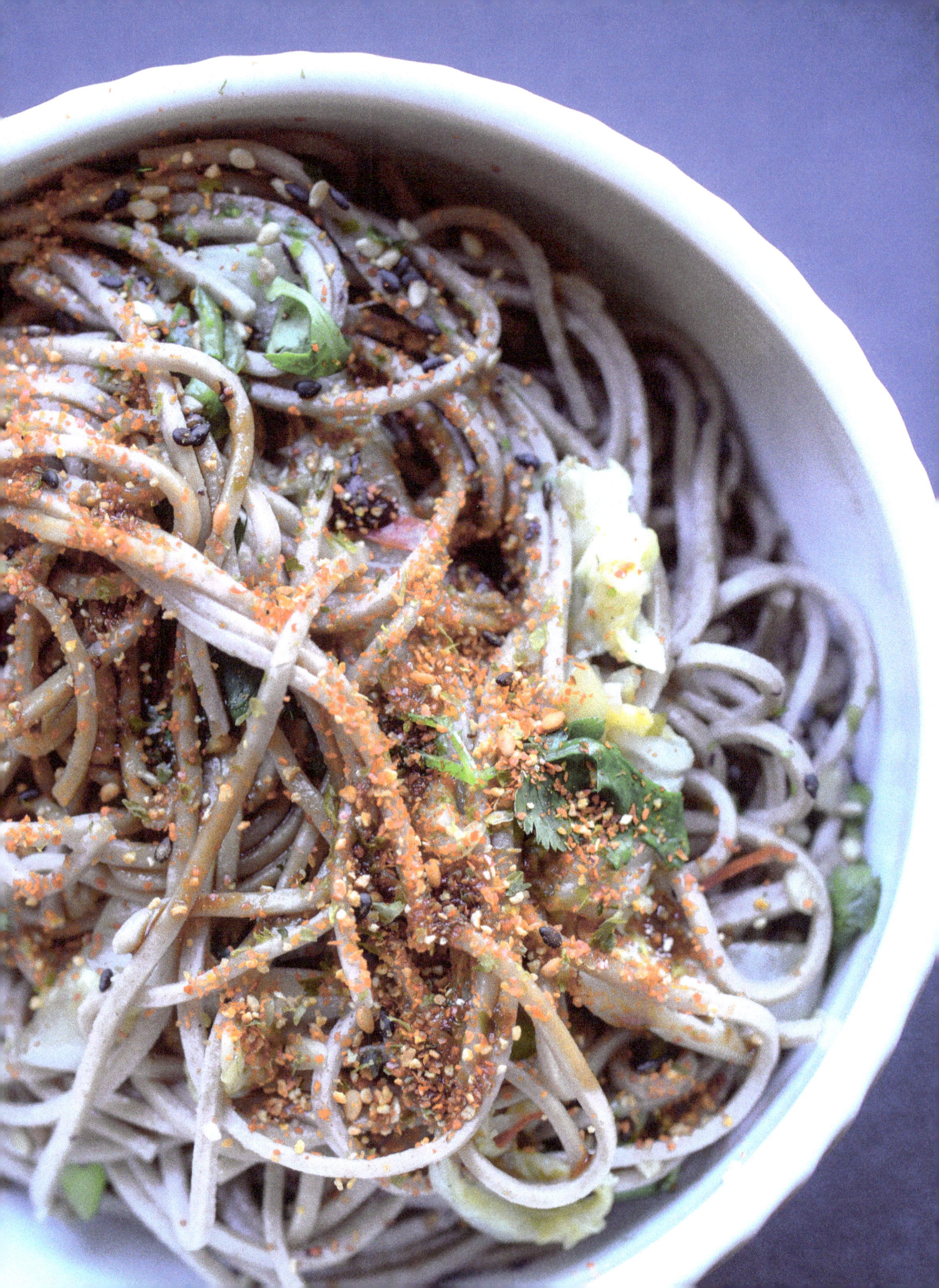

SOBA NOODLE STIR FRY

SERVES 4

125 g	Shiitake mushrooms, fresh OR 8 shiitake mushrooms, dried
250–300 g	Soba noodles
1 tbsp	Sesame oil
Pinch	Sea salt
1 tbsp	Ginger, grated
2 tsp	Garlic, minced
1–2	Chillies
2 cups	Chinese cabbage (wombok), sliced, or bok choy, stems sliced diagonally into 2 cm strips and leaves sliced diagonally into 5 cm strips
2	Spring onions, chopped
2 tbsp	Mirin
2 tbsp	Tamari or shoyu
2 tbsp	Coriander, chopped
1–2 tsp	Sesame seeds, toasted or sea vegetable seasoning (I use Furikake seasoning from Spiral Foods)

- If using fresh shiitake: Remove stems and cut caps into 2 cm slices.
- If using dried shiitake: Soak shiitake mushrooms for at least 30 minutes in 5 cups warm water from the kettle (see tip on p.16) or for even better flavour, soak overnight. Strain and keep soaking water. Discard stems and slice shiitake caps.
- Boil 2 litres of water in a large pot then gently add soba noodles (see tip below). Simmer for about 3 minutes. (Don't overcook as noodles will be added to stir fry for more cooking.)
- While noodles are cooking, heat oil in a large wok, add shiitake mushrooms and sea salt. Sauté over medium heat for 1 minute, then add ginger, garlic, chillies and slices of Chinese cabbage or stems of bok choy.
  Add 3–4 tbsp of shiitake soaking water or water.
- Sauté for 1 minute, then, if using, add bok choy leaves, and continue to sauté until both the leaves and stems are tender, about 1–2 minutes more. You can add more Chinese cabbage if you are using that.
- Reduce heat and add spring onions, mirin and tamari. Quickly stir in pre-cooked soba noodles and chopped coriander. Adjust seasoning to taste.
- Sprinkle with sesame seeds or seasoning and serve warm or at room temperature.

TIP FOR COOKING SOBA NOODLES

Bring 2 litres of water to boil and add noodles little by little to stop them from clumping together. Add 1 cup cold water. When water returns to the boil, add another cup of cold water. When it boils again, add 1 more cup of cold water and simmer – do not boil – until noodles are softened but still firm. Drain then rinse in cold water.

Ideal cooking times are 3 minutes for stir fries and 4 minutes for soups and salads.

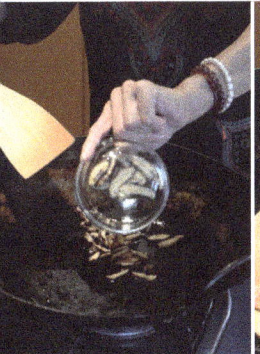 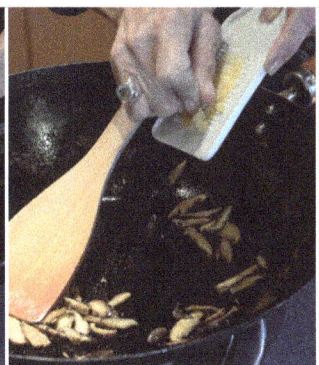 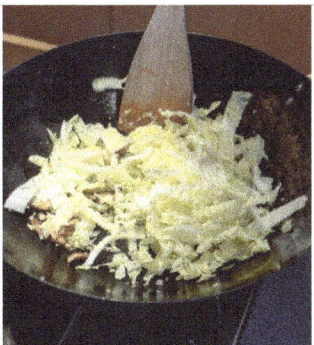 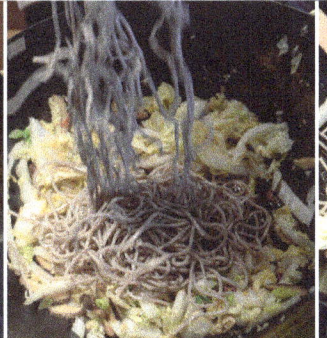 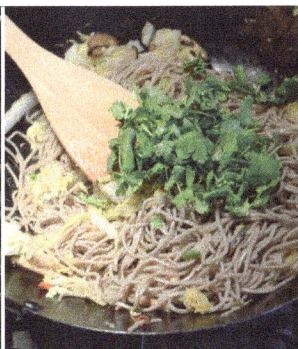

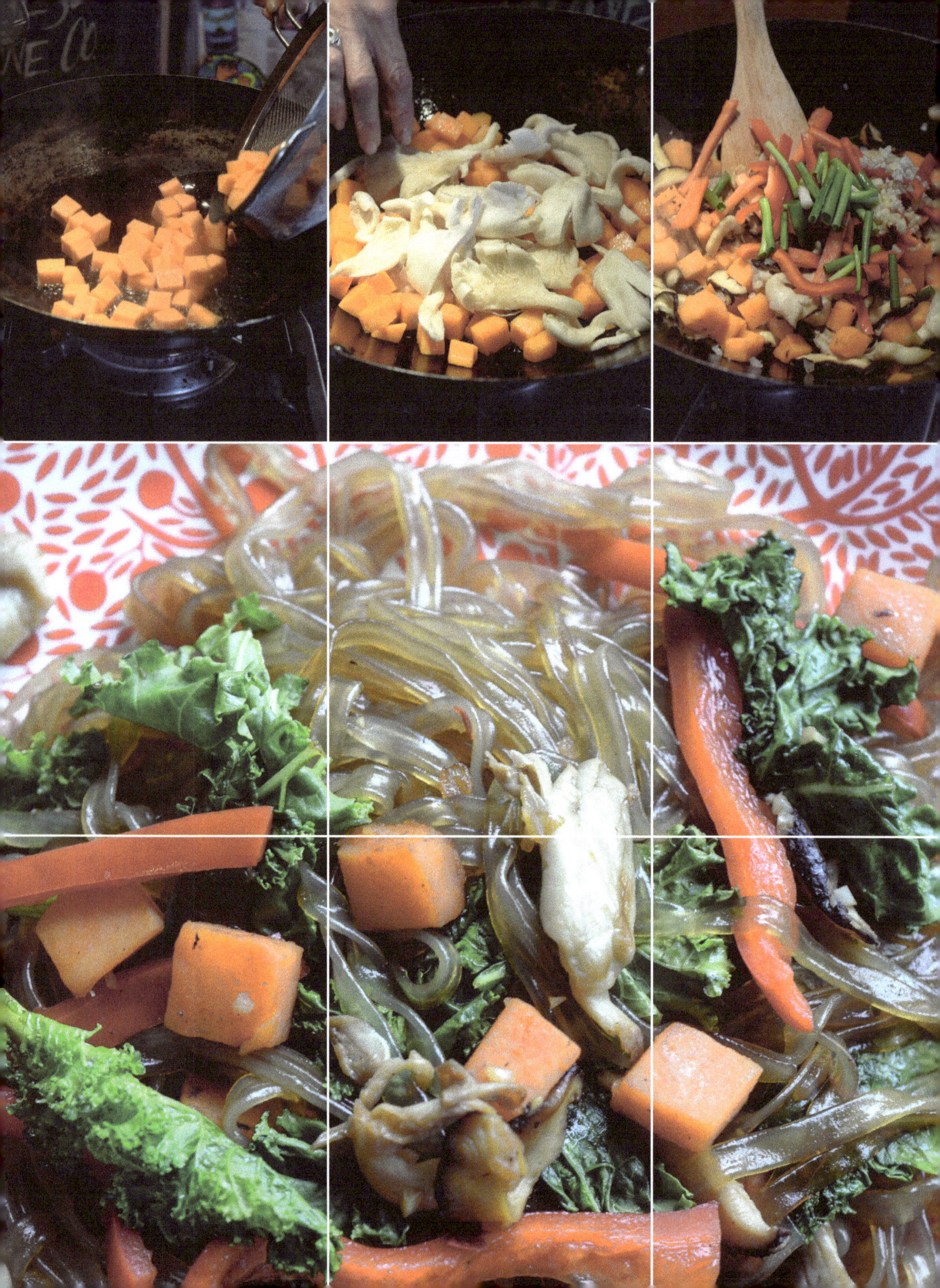

SWEET POTATO NOODLE STIR FRY

SERVES 4

300 g	Sweet potato noodles
Pinch	Sea salt
2 tbsp	Coconut oil
2 cups	Sweet potato, small diced
100 g	Oyster mushrooms, fresh
100 g	Shiitake mushrooms, fresh
1 large	Shallot, chopped
½	Red capsicum, cut into strips
2 cloves	Garlic, chopped
3	Spring onions, 3 cm pieces
6 leaves	Kale, stems discarded and leaves chopped
Garnish	Sesame seeds, toasted (use black sesame seeds for a tasty change)

SAUCE

¼ cup	Coconut or rice syrup
⅓ cup	Tamari or shoyu
1 tbsp	Mirin
1 tbsp	Toasted sesame oil
1 tbsp	Ginger, grated

- In a small bowl, combine sauce ingredients and whisk together. Set aside.
- Bring a large pot of water to boil. Add sea salt and stir in noodles. Simmer for about 6 minutes. (Don't overcook noodles as they are cooked again in wok.)
- Drain then rinse with cold water. Set aside.
- Heat coconut oil in a large wok. On medium heat, add sweet potato and fry for 4 minutes before turning and frying for a further 4 minutes. Sweet potato cubes should be lightly browned, a darker orange and just nearly cooked through.
- Add oyster and shiitake mushrooms and stir fry for about 5 minutes.
- Add chopped shallot and a pinch of sea salt and stir fry for about 2 minutes.
- Add sliced red capsicum, garlic and spring onions, reduce heat and stir fry for an extra minute or until red capsicum is starting to soften.
- Add sliced kale and pre-cooked noodles and stir fry for another few minutes.
- Add sauce and toss through.
- Sprinkle with toasted sesame seeds to serve.

This was inspired by a tasty Korean Japchae I had in a restaurant.

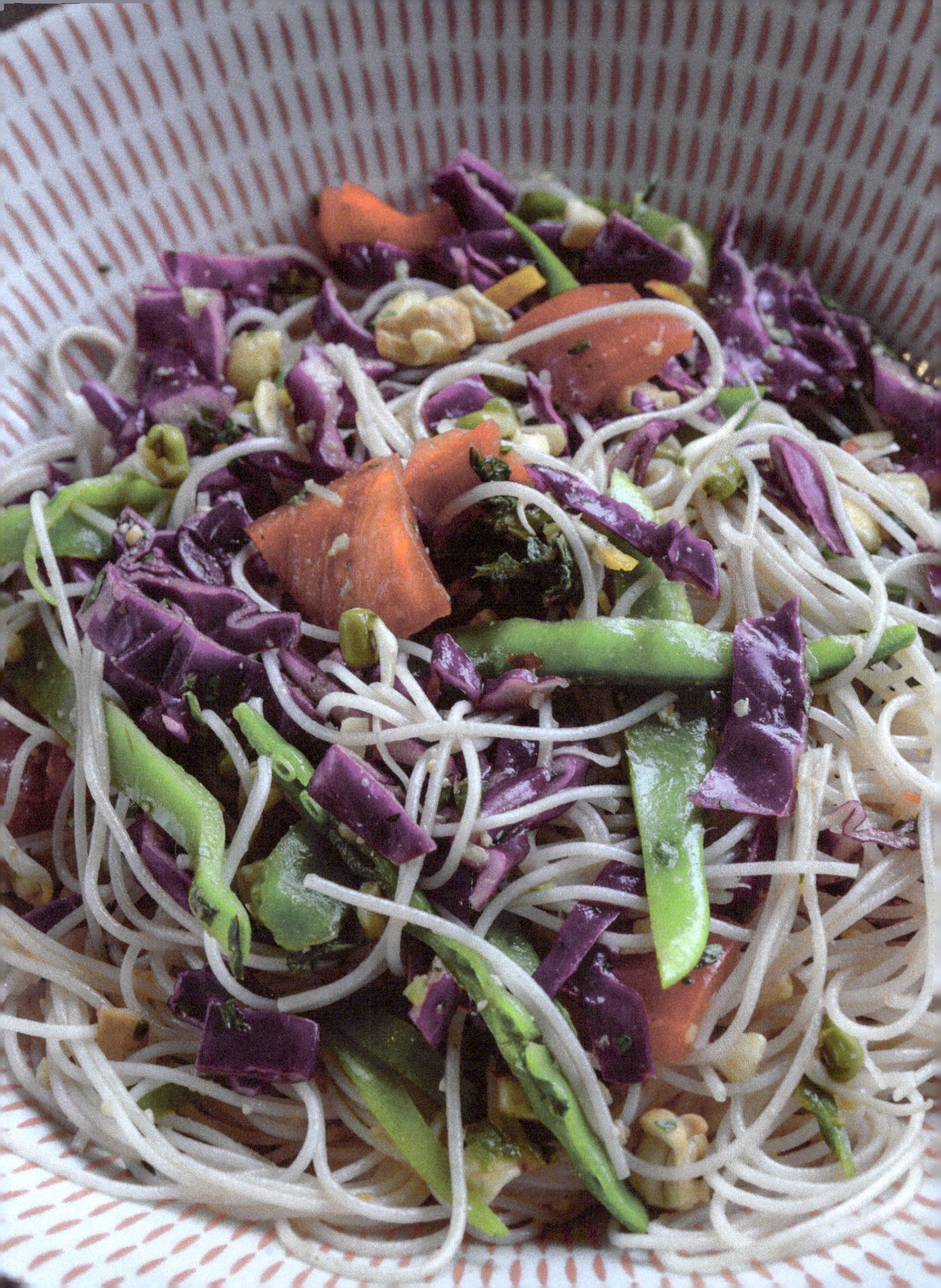

RICE OR BEAN NOODLE SALAD

SERVES 4

150–200 g	Rice or bean noodles
1 cup	Red cabbage, shredded
10	Snow peas, blanched and sliced
1 small	Red capsicum, sliced
100 g	Sprouts, any type (e.g. mung bean)
To taste	Tamari or shoyu
½ cup	Cashews, roasted and chopped

DRESSING

1 tsp	Ginger, grated
2	Garlic cloves
3 tbsp	Orange zest
15 sprigs	Coriander leaves, stems removed
2	Spring onions
5 tbsp	Apple cider vinegar
¼ cup	Toasted sesame oil
1 tbsp	Maple, coconut or rice syrup
1 tsp	Chilli (I use organic minced chilli)
1 tsp	Sea salt

- Prepare noodles per packet instructions. Drain thoroughly and place in salad bowl.
- Toss in cabbage, snow peas, capsicum and sprouts.
- In a food processor, prepare the dressing by blending all of the dressing ingredients.
- Pour the dressing over the noodles and toss.
- Add tamari to taste.
- Garnish with chopped roasted cashews.

VARIATION: Add cooked tempeh or tofu.

I used Bifun Rice Noodles for this photo

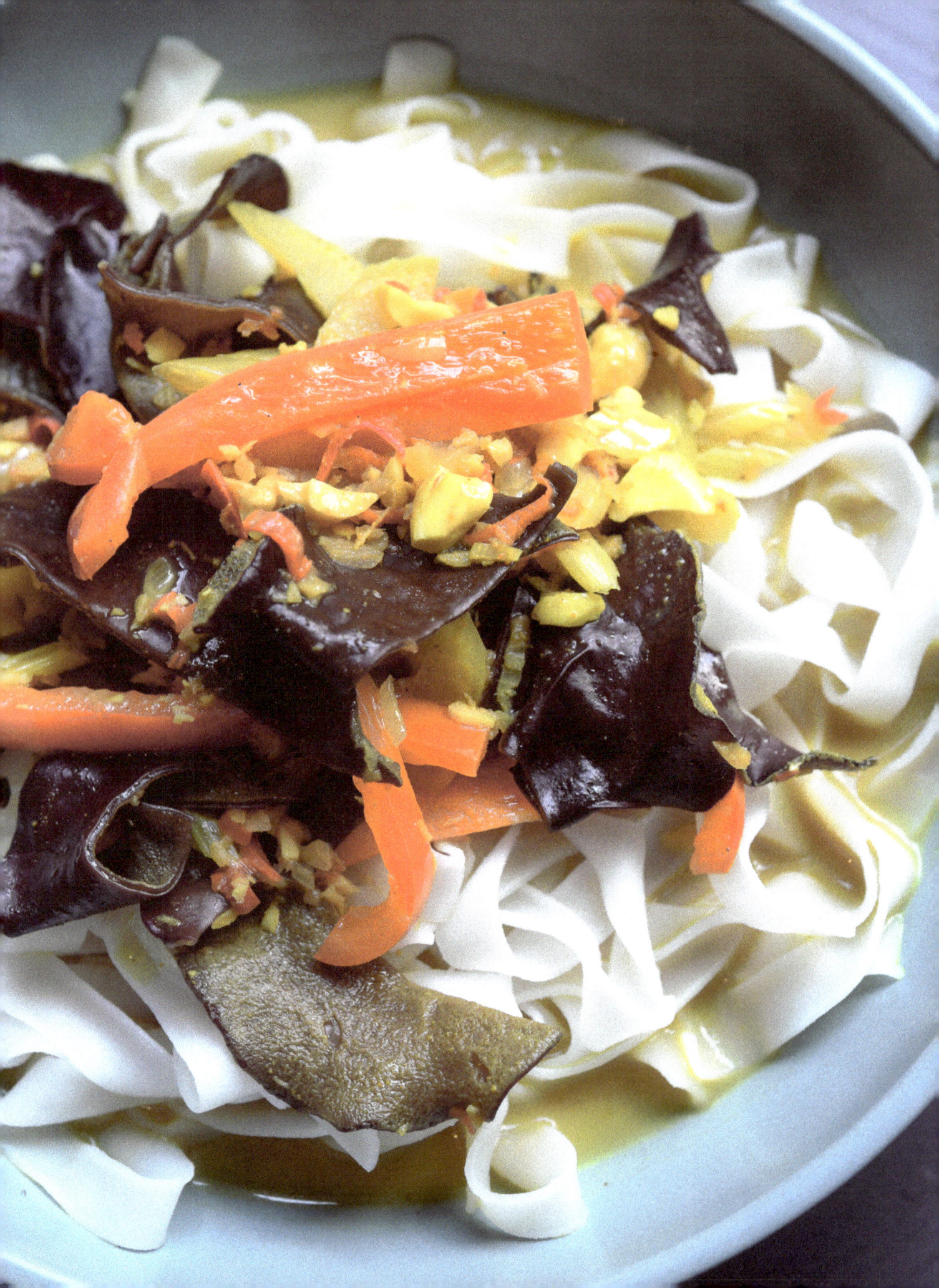

CHIANG MAI VEGETABLE NOODLES

SERVES 3–4

200 g	Flat rice noodles
1 tbsp	Coconut oil
2 cloves	Garlic, sliced
2 tbsp	Red curry paste (see recipe p.43)
½–1 tsp	Dried chillies, crushed (optional)
250 ml	Coconut milk
500 ml	Thai vegetable stock
¼ tsp	Turmeric powder
2 tsp	Curry powder
2 tbsp	Tamari or shoyu (or you can use sea salt instead)
15 g	Coconut sugar
2 stalks	Celery, sliced
25 g	Shallots, chopped
1 small	Red capsicum
25 g	Wood ear mushrooms (fresh or dried)
4 tbsp	Roasted cashews, crushed
2–3 tbsp	Lime juice

I was fortunate to be a student at cooking classes in Thailand and this is my vegetarian version of a recipe that included chicken. Prepare Thai stock first (see recipe p.17)

- Prepare noodles per packet instructions then drain and rinse in cold water.
- Heat wok, add oil, and then stir in garlic.
- Add curry paste and dried chillies, if desired, and mix well.
- Pour in coconut milk, stirring continuously, then bring to the boil and cook until the liquid thickens a little.
- Add Thai vegetable stock, turmeric, curry powder, tamari or shoyu or salt and coconut sugar and bring back to the boil.
- Lower heat and add sliced celery, chopped shallots, sliced capsicum, sliced mushrooms and roasted cashews.
- Bring back to the boil and then remove from the heat.
- To serve, put the noodles in a large serving bowl and pour the wok mix over them.
- Sprinkle with lime juice to taste.

TIP: If you can't buy fresh wood ear mushrooms, buy dried and soak to soften before adding into this recipe.

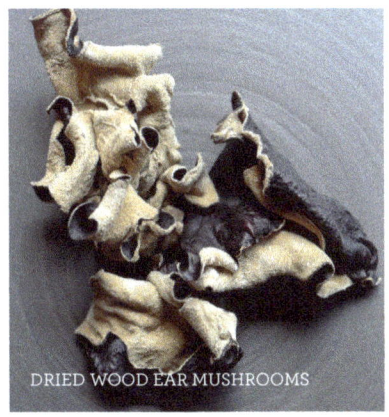

DRIED WOOD EAR MUSHROOMS

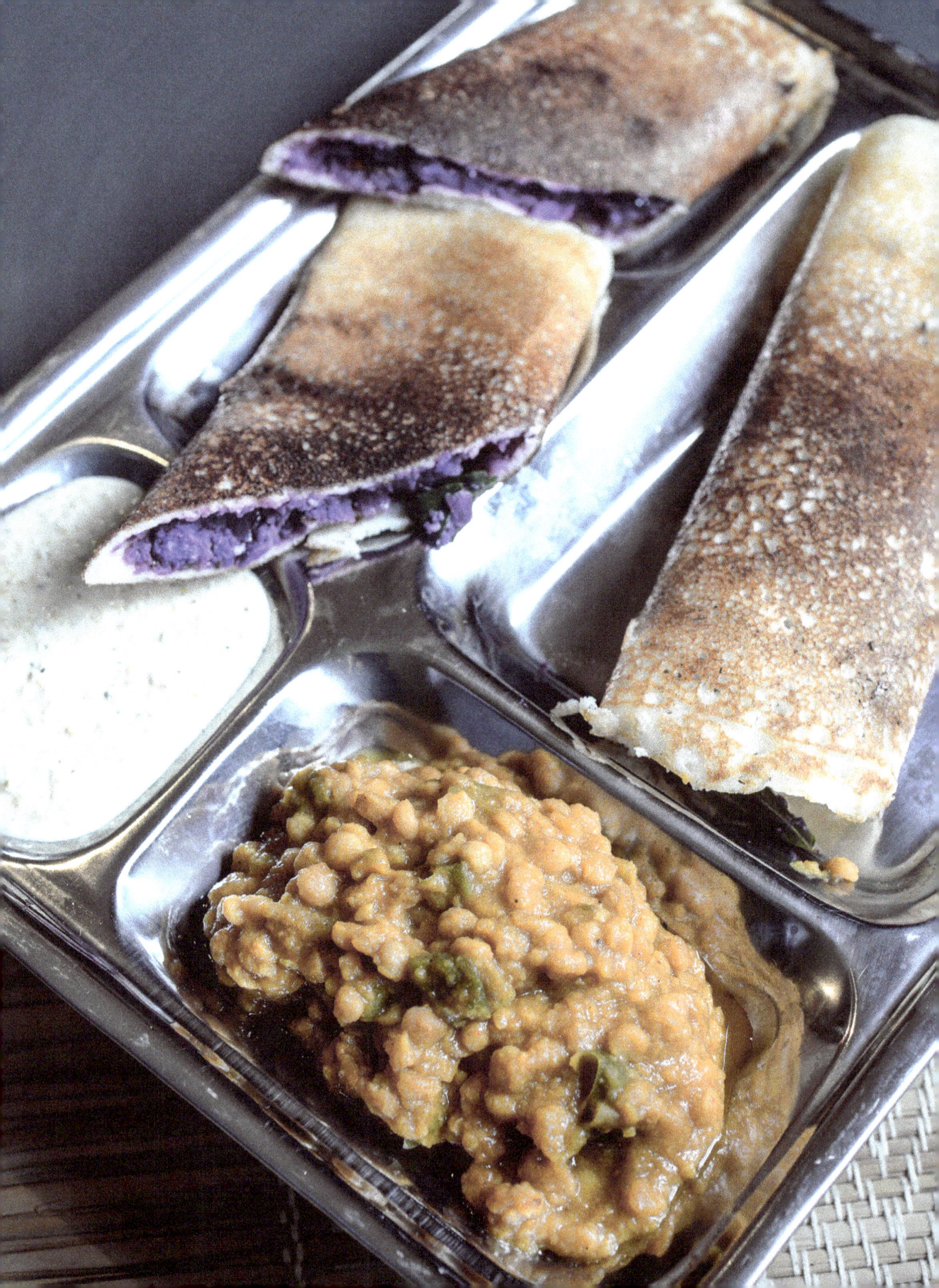

MWC Specials

Sandy's Seed Mix 124

Kukicha Twig Tea 124

Plain Dosa 125

Masala Dosa 127

Coconut Chutney 127

Corn Tortillas And Taco Shells 128

SANDY'S SEED MIX

MAKES 2 CUPS
KEEPS WELL FOR ONE WEEK

1 cup	Sunflower seeds
1 cup	Pumpkin (pepita) seeds
1 tbsp	Tamari or Worcestershire sauce (Melrose Health makes a tasty gluten-free Worcestershire sauce)

- Preheat oven to 150°C.
- Place seeds onto a baking tray and toast in oven about 15 minutes.
- Remove seeds from oven and switch off oven.
- Add tamari or Worcestershire sauce to seeds and mix through.
- Place back into still-warm oven for 5 minutes.
- Remove to cool.
- Place seasoned seeds into a jar and cool before closing with the lid.

KUKICHA TWIG TEA

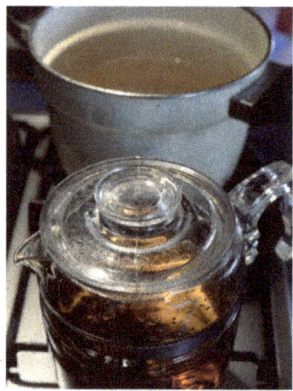

Since my very first cooking class, I have served Kukicha twig tea in a heat-resistant glass pot (remember the old coffee percolators of the 1970s?). This is only my third of these pots – I remember both times when I broke the other two. I actually found my current pot in an op shop (charity shop). Thousands of cups of this tea have been served in all my classes and to all my friends too.

The world of Japanese green tea is vast, with literally thousands of varieties, each featuring subtle differences in taste and aroma.

Kukicha is Japanese for twig tea. It's made only from the twigs and stems of the green tea plant.

Kukicha tea is low in stimulants. It is roasted in cast-iron cauldrons to lessen its bitterness and to decrease the tannins. It is favoured among Macrobiotics, as it contains almost no caffeine.

According to Macrobiotics, twig tea is a digestive aid; it helps to neutralise an overly acidic digestive system because it is high in minerals and low in caffeine. Because twig tea comprises the stems and young twigs, it is rich in both the vitamins and minerals that feed the growth parts of the plant. The minerals found in Kukicha include copper, selenium, manganese, calcium, zinc and fluoride. Kukicha also contains vitamins A and C and the B-complex vitamins, which are all potent antioxidants. According to The Everything Guide to Macrobiotics, by Julie Ong, Kukicha has an alkalising effect and lowers acidity.

Kukicha does not overly stimulate and therefore can be consumed many times per day.

TO MAKE THE TEA

- Simmer twig tea for up to 20 minutes in glass a heat-resistant pot or saucepan to give it body, a deep flavour, more available nutrients and to make it a more warming drink.
- For a more cooling beverage, you can steep it for 5 minutes.

CAFFEINE CONTENT COMPARISON

Approximate caffeine content per 250 ml cup

Coffee	150–200 mg
Black tea	70–100 mg
Cola	45 mg
Sencha green tea	12 mg
Kukicha twig tea	7 mg

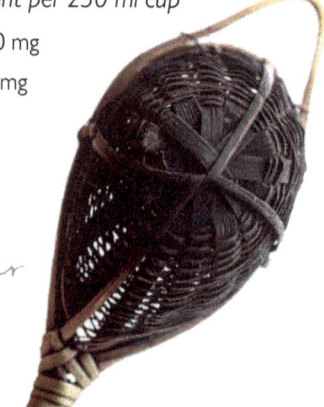

My favourite bamboo tea strainer

TIP: DOSA

Dosa is a fermented crepe made from rice batter and black lentils. It is a common breakfast dish, street food and a staple dish in the south Indian states of Karnataka, Tamil Nadu, Telangana, Andhra Pradesh and Kerala. It is also popular in other parts of India and other countries like Sri Lanka, Mauritius, Myanmar, Nepal, Malaysia and Singapore.

As its constituent ingredients are rice and urad dal (skinned black lentils), it is a good source of protein.

The fermentation process increases the vitamin B and C content.

The plain dosa recipe calls for soaking urad dal and rice. The soaked lentils and rice are then finely ground and fermented overnight. A warm temperature is important for the batter to ferment well.

When cooking, it's best to use a griddle, flat cast-iron skillet or plate, or dosa pan.

PLAIN DOSA

MAKES ABOUT 15 DOSA
THIS BATTER KEEPS REFRIGERATED FOR UP TO 1 WEEK

300 g	Short-grain rice (known as idli rice)
100 g	Urad dal, split and washed
1 tsp	Fenugreek seeds (optional)
Pinch	Sea salt
For frying	Natural sesame oil (vegetable oil is OK but coconut oil is too heavy)

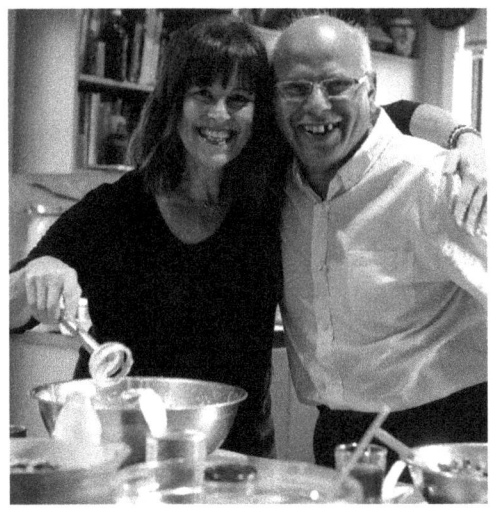

- Wash rice then wash dal with fenugreek seeds and soak separately for at least 4 hours (overnight is best). Drain.
- In food processor or by hand, grind rice coarsely. Add 1 cup water.
- In food processor or by hand, grind dal–fenugreek mix to a smooth and fluffy consistency, adding ½ cup water.
- Mix together and leave to ferment overnight.
- Add sea salt and extra warm water to make a pouring consistency.
- Heat the dosa pan, griddle or skillet and grease lightly with sesame oil (don't use toasted sesame oil as it is too rich in sesame flavour).
- Pour out a spoonful of batter and spread to form a round about 10 cm in diameter.
- Cook for 2 minutes. Turn over and cook for another 1 or 2 minutes.
- Serve dosa hot with coconut chutney (see recipe p.127) and slow cooked curried dahl (see recipe p.107) or a *sambar.

*Sambar, also spelt sambhar, is a lentil-based vegetable stew or chowder based around a broth made with tamarind.

Thanks to my good friend Master Chef Jitendra Bhatia for sharing this recipe with me.

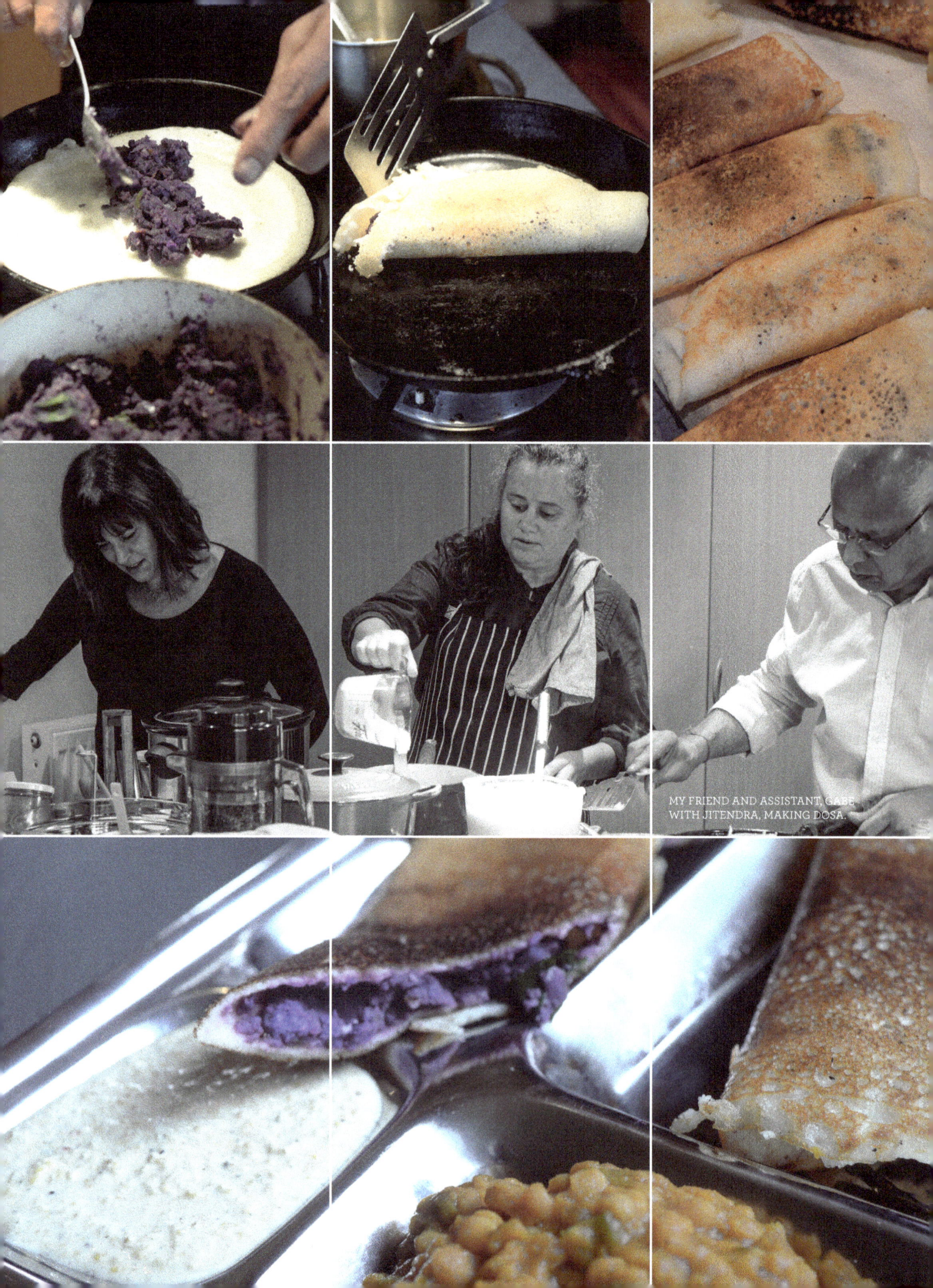

MY FRIEND AND ASSISTANT, GABE WITH JITENDRA, MAKING DOSA.

Masala dosa is plain dosa filled with potato, mustard seeds and curry leaves.

MASALA DOSA

MAKES ENOUGH FILLING FOR ABOUT 8 DOSA

1 quantity	Plain dosa, cooked (see recipe p123)
3 tbsp	Ghee or coconut oil
1 tsp	Mustard seeds
½ tsp	Cumin seeds
2 small	Red chillies, dried, chopped
1 medium	Onion, diced
½ tsp	Sea salt
½ tsp	Turmeric, ground
Pinch	Asafoetida (optional)
1 tbsp	Ginger, grated
10	Curry leaves (you can remove leaves or throw in whole sprigs of leaves still attached to their branches and then retrieve before serving)
4 cloves	Garlic, minced
2 small	Green chillies, finely chopped
700 g	Potatoes, boiled, peeled and cubed (see tip)
½ cup	Coriander, leaves and tender stems roughly chopped

- Put ghee or oil in pan over medium heat. When oil is warm add mustard and cumin seeds. Wait for seeds to pop, about 1 minute, then add dried red chilli and onion.
- Cook, stirring, until onions have softened, about 5 minutes.
- Season lightly with sea salt and add turmeric, asafoetida, ginger, curry leaves, garlic and green chilli. Stir to coat and fry for 1 more minute.
- Add potato and ½ cup water. Cook, stirring well to combine, until liquid has evaporated, about 5 minutes.
- Roughly mash potato mixture. Season well with extra salt, add chopped coriander, and then set aside.
- Spread the potato filling on one side of the pre-made dosa. Cover with the other half and let dosa cook for 15 to 30 seconds to heat through.
- Serve dosa hot with coconut chutney and slow cooked sweet potato curried dahl (see recipe p123) or a *sambar.

TIP: *Make sure the potatoes you choose are good for mashing and are dry. I use the Purple Congo as it is a member of the healthy sweet potato family, good for mashing and purple ... different from traditional white potatoes!*

*Sambar, also spelled sambhar, is a lentil-based vegetable stew or chowder based around a broth made with tamarind. It's not made in this book.

COCONUT CHUTNEY

MAKES ABOUT 3 CUPS
KEEP REFRIGERATED FOR UP TO 1 WEEK

30 g	Chana dal
1 ½ tsp	Coconut oil
1 tsp	Black mustard seeds
10 g	Red chilli, dried
10 g	Curry leaves
115 g	Coconut, grated or shredded (organic is best)
500 ml	Coconut milk
Pinch	Sea salt, to taste
½	Lime or lemon juice

- Soak chana dal in water for ½ hour. Drain.
- Heat oil in a small frypan or saucepan over medium heat and, just before it starts to smoke, add mustard seeds. Cover and cook until mustard seeds begin to crackle, 1 to 2 minutes.
- Add drained chana dal and red chilli and cook until they start to brown, then add curry leaves (this will cause the oil to splatter so be careful).
- Add coconut and fry for 1 minute more, until slightly brown.
- Remove ingredients from pan and using a mortar and pestle, blender or food processor, grind or blend to a smooth paste.
- Add coconut milk and mix well.
- Add sea salt and lime or lemon juice to taste.

CORN TORTILLAS AND TACO SHELLS

MAKES 12

2 cups	Masa harina (tortilla flour)
1 cup	Water
2 tsp	Sea salt

TO MAKE THE DOUGH

- Combine masa harina with water.
- Mix with hands until dough is moist but holds its shape, adding more water if needed.
- Let dough rest for 15 minutes.
- Divide dough into 12 balls and dampen slightly with water.
- Using a tortilla press or a flat baking dish, press dough between two pieces of baking paper to make a 12 cm round.
- Repeat until all dough balls have been used.

TO MAKE TORTILLAS

- Carefully peel off the top sheet of paper and place tortilla, paper side up, on a hot ungreased griddle or skillet.
- Gently peel off remaining paper.
- Cook for 30 seconds or until edges begin to dry.
- Turn and cook until surface appears puffy.
- Repeat with remaining rounds.

TO MAKE TACO SHELLS

- In a heavy skillet heat $\frac{2}{3}$ cm cooking oil.
- Remove tortilla round from paper and fry for 10 seconds or until limp.
- With tongs, fold tortilla in half. Continue frying for 1 minute, or until crisp, turning once. Hold edges apart at all times.
- Drain on paper towel.
- Repeat with remaining rounds.

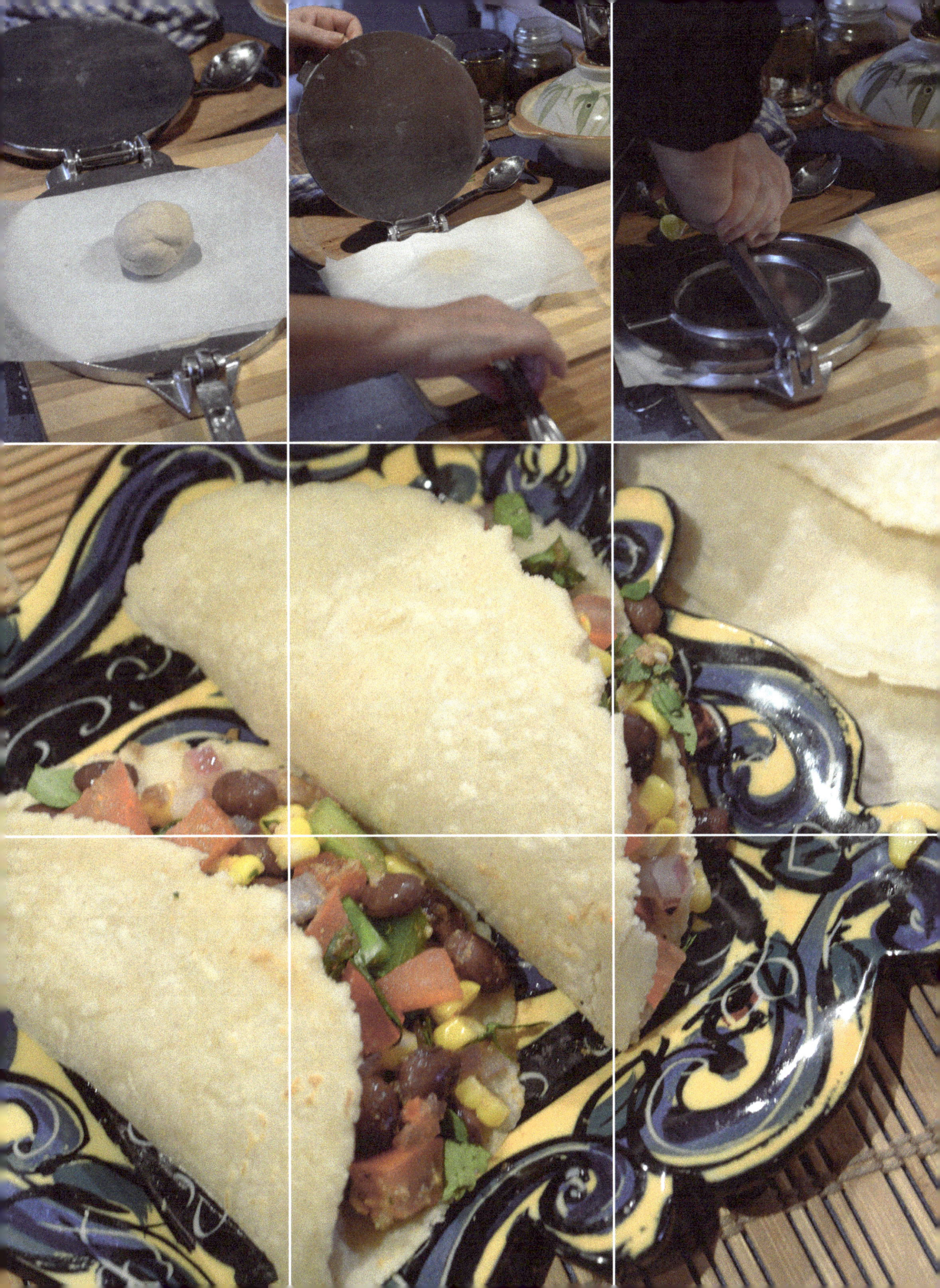

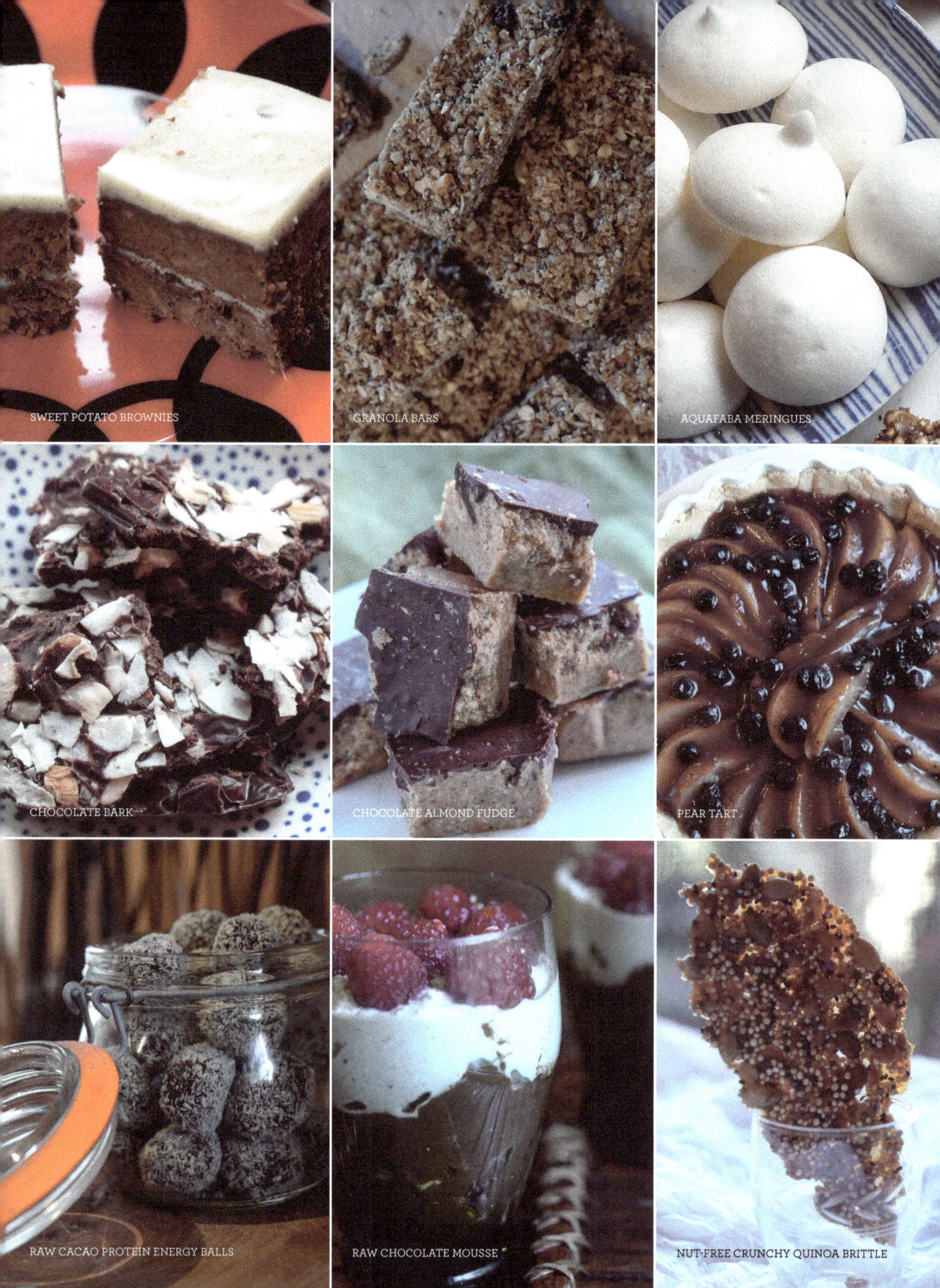

Sweet Treats

Homemade Nut Mylk 132

Sweet Potato Brownies 133

Coconut Buttercream Icing 133

Ginger Chocolate Chip Cookies 134

Ginger Apple Pear Sauce 134

Raw Chocolate Mousse 135

Chocolate Almond Fudge 135

Granola Bars 136

Chocolate Bark 139

Nut-Free Crunchy Quinoa Brittle 141

Panforte Slice 141

Pear Tart 142

Aquafaba Meringues 144

Raw Cacao Protein Energy Balls 145

Homemade Chocolate 145

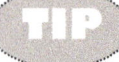 **ABOUT MYLK**

Mylk is the term used to describe non-dairy milk products (like from soy, almonds, coconuts, peanuts, cashew, hemp, sesame) and clearly distinguishes it from the common understanding of milk.

Many raw food recipes call for nut mylk. These mylks are delicious on their own, in smoothies, with a breakfast cereal or spiced with a bit of cinnamon and nutmeg. If you'd like to try nut mylk as a non-dairy substitute, here's how to make it.

It's so easy and far more economical than paying for packaged mylks at health foods stores and supermarkets. Think about all the added oils and filler ingredients that you don't need to be drinking!

I like almonds and cashews but you can use hazelnuts, walnuts and other nuts too.

You'll need a fine strainer or a nut mylk bag for this recipe. You can buy these at health food stores, or you can make your own.

HOMEMADE NUT MYLK

MAKES 1 LITRE
LASTS UP TO 3 DAYS IN REFRIGERATOR

| 1 cup | Nuts |
| 4 cups | Water (alkalised filtered water tastes best) |

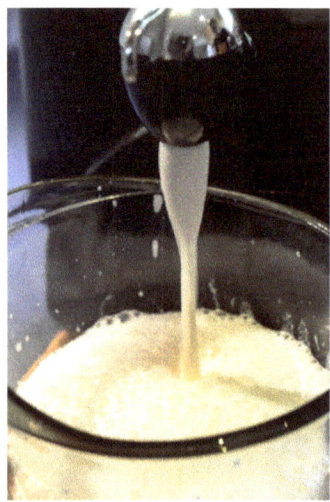

- Soak 1 cup of nuts in water to cover for at least 5 hours (though overnight is best).
- Once soaked, rinse nuts well and drain.
- Put the drained nuts into a high-powered blender with 4 cups of filtered water and blend well.
- Use a fine strainer or nut mylk bag to remove pulp if desired. I like to use the mylk without straining.

VARIATIONS: For a sweeter taste, add some pre-soaked dates, honey, seeds of a vanilla bean pod or vanilla powder to the blender.

You can use more or less water to vary the thickness of your raw nut mylk, depending on your personal preference, but in general, you want a 1:4 ratio of nuts to water. Please experiment.

SWEET POTATO BROWNIES
With Coconut Buttercream Icing

STORE IN REFRIGERATOR OR FREEZER

2 cups	Sweet potato, peeled and chopped
1 cup	Nut butter (I like almond or cashew butter)
4 tbsp	Coconut or maple syrup
½ cup	Raw cacao powder
1 tsp	Cinnamon, ground
1 tsp	Vanilla powder (use organic vanilla bean powder)
4 tbsp	Orange zest, grated
⅓ cup	Carob or cacao nibs (optional)
	Coconut oil to grease cake pan

I use a 15 x 15 cm baking pan.

- Steam peeled, chopped sweet potato until softened, then mash.
- Preheat the oven to 180°C and grease your cake pan.
- In a saucepan, melt nut butter with syrup.
- In a large bowl, add mashed sweet potato, nut butter mixture, cacao powder, cinnamon, vanilla and orange zest and mix well.
- Fold in carob or cacao nibs (if using).
- Pour mixture into greased pan and bake for 20 minutes or until cooked through.
- Remove from the oven and allow to cool completely before adding icing. See recipe below.
- Spread the icing in a thick layer over the top of the cooled brownies. It will be quite soft so carefully use a knife to spread the icing to the edge of the cake. The icing will firm up within 15–20 minutes of being left undisturbed.
- Slice into squares or bars.

COCONUT BUTTERCREAM ICING

MAKES 2 CUPS

1 ½ cups	Coconut butter
½ cup	Coconut or maple syrup
1 tsp	Vanilla, powder
1 tbsp	Lemon zest
3–4 tbsp	Water (I always prefer to use alkalised filtered water... it tastes best)

- In a high-powered blender or food processor, combine coconut butter, syrup, vanilla and lemon zest and blend at high speed, stopping if you need to scrape down the sides, until smooth.
- Add water 1 tbsp at a time until icing reaches your desired consistency.
- Use immediately.

These ginger choc chip cookies are tasty, tangy and really moist.

GINGER CHOCOLATE CHIP COOKIES

MAKES ABOUT 12-15
THESE CAN BE STORED IN AN AIRTIGHT CONTAINER IN THE REFRIGERATOR FOR 1 WEEK

3 cups	Almond flour
½ tsp	Sea salt
½ tsp	Baking soda
½ cup	Pecans or other nuts, chopped (optional)
½ cup	Chocolate chips (naturally sweetened)
½ cup	Ginger apple pear sauce (see recipe below)
½ cup	Rice syrup
1 tsp	Ginger juice (grate ginger then squeeze out juice)
1 tbsp	Vanilla extract

- Preheat oven to 150°C and line a tray with baking paper.
- Combine dry ingredients in a large bowl and wet ingredients in a smaller bowl.
- Mix wet ingredients into dry.
- Pinch off pieces of mixture and form into small balls (4–5 cm). Place on the baking tray and press to flatten a little.
- Bake for 10 minutes.
- Cool and serve.

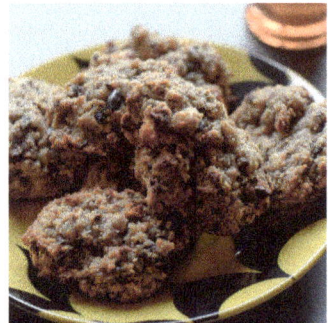

GINGER APPLE PEAR SAUCE

KEEPS REFRIGERATED IN A GLASS JAR FOR UP TO 1 WEEK

4	Apples
4	Pears
Pinch	Sea salt
2 tsp	Ginger juice (grate ginger then squeeze out juice)

- Wash fruit, remove the cores, peel and then slice into bite-sized pieces.
- Place in a pot with a little water and add a pinch of sea salt. Simmer on a very low heat until the fruit is soft, approximately 10 minutes. Remove from heat.
- Blend to a cream using an upright blender or a stick blender. Squeeze in fresh ginger juice to taste.
- Serve with almond cream, chopped seeds or nuts, or porridge, or enjoy on its own.

Delicious as dessert and used in ginger chocolate chip cookies recipe. As always, using organic fruit tastes best.

RAW CHOCOLATE MOUSSE

SERVES 2 (OR 3, IF YOU EAT LESS – NOT EASY TO DO)

1 tsp	Coconut oil
1	Avocado
1 tsp	Water
2 tbsp	Raw cacao powder
2 tbsp	Coconut or rice syrup (rice syrup gives a more butterscotch flavour)
1 tsp	Cardamom, ground
1 cup	Berries (raspberries, blueberries, blackberries etc.)
Garnish	Mint leaves
Garnish	Almonds, crushed

- Melt coconut oil.
- Place melted coconut oil, avocado and water into a blender or food processor and blend until smooth, adding a little more water if required.
- Add cacao powder, syrup and cardamom and blend again until smooth.
- Taste and adjust sweetness as desired.
- Serve with berries and garnish with chopped mint leaves and crushed almonds.
- A tasty tip is to add nut cream (see recipe p.149)

CHOCOLATE ALMOND FUDGE

SERVES 15-20
KEEP IN FREEZER

1 cup	Almond butter
4 tbsp	Coconut oil
2 tbsp	Maple syrup
½ tsp	Sea salt
100 g	Dark chocolate

I use a 15 x 15 cm baking tin.

- In a small saucepan over low heat, mix almond butter, coconut oil, maple syrup and salt until smooth. Remove from heat.
- Line a baking tin with baking paper and pour in mixture. Spread with a wet spatula.
- Melt chopped dark chocolate in a double saucepan then spread on top of mixture. Freeze for at least 2 hours.
- Remove tin from freezer then carefully remove fudge by lifting the ends of the baking paper.
- Cut into 2 cm squares and store in freezer, separating each layer with baking paper.

GRANOLA BARS

MAKES 14–16 9 X 4 CM BARS
THESE KEEP WELL IN AN AIRTIGHT CONTAINER IN THE
REFRIGERATOR FOR 1 WEEK

230 g	Rolled oats (organic or biodynamic tastes best)
120 g	Almonds, roasted
120 g	Pumpkin seeds, roasted
30 g	Chia seeds
120 g	Goji berries, currants or any dried berries
½ tsp	Cinnamon, ground
170 ml	Maple syrup (or any other liquid sweetener)
100 ml	Honey
2 tsp	Extra virgin olive oil
1 tsp	Vanilla extract or powder (organic tastes best)
Pinch	Sea salt

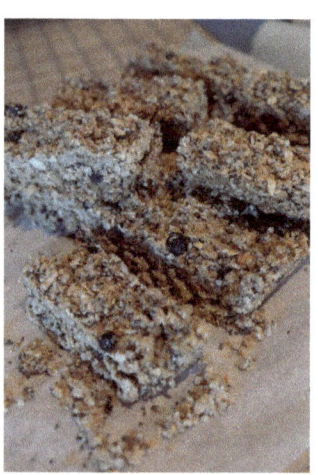

I use my porcelain baking tray, which measures 27 x 18 cm and is 6 cm deep.

- Preheat oven to 180°C then place oats onto baking tray to roast for several minutes until they release a nutty fragrance and begin to brown slightly (you can also roast almonds and pumpkin seeds at the same time.) Remove oats and place them in a large mixing bowl. Allow to cool.
- Reduce oven to 150°C.
- Place roasted almonds in food processor and pulse several seconds until coarsely ground. Pour into the bowl of oats.
- Pulse roasted pumpkin seeds for 2 to 3 seconds and add to the bowl.
- Place all dried fruit in the bowl then mix all ingredients thoroughly.
- Place syrup, honey and oil in a medium saucepan and bring to the boil. Reduce the heat to medium and simmer, stirring constantly, for 5 minutes. As the syrup cooks, it will begin to thicken.
- Add ground cinnamon, sea salt and vanilla to the syrup mix. Continue stirring for 2 more minutes. Remove from heat.
- Pour the syrup blend over the oat mixture and mix well to coat ingredients.
- Lightly oil a baking tray and line with baking paper. Moisten hands very lightly and firmly press the oat mixture into the tray. Spread it evenly to about 5 cm in height.
- Place in the pre-heated oven and bake for about 30 minutes or until light golden brown.
- Remove from the oven and let cool for about 2 hours to harden.
- Slice into bars.

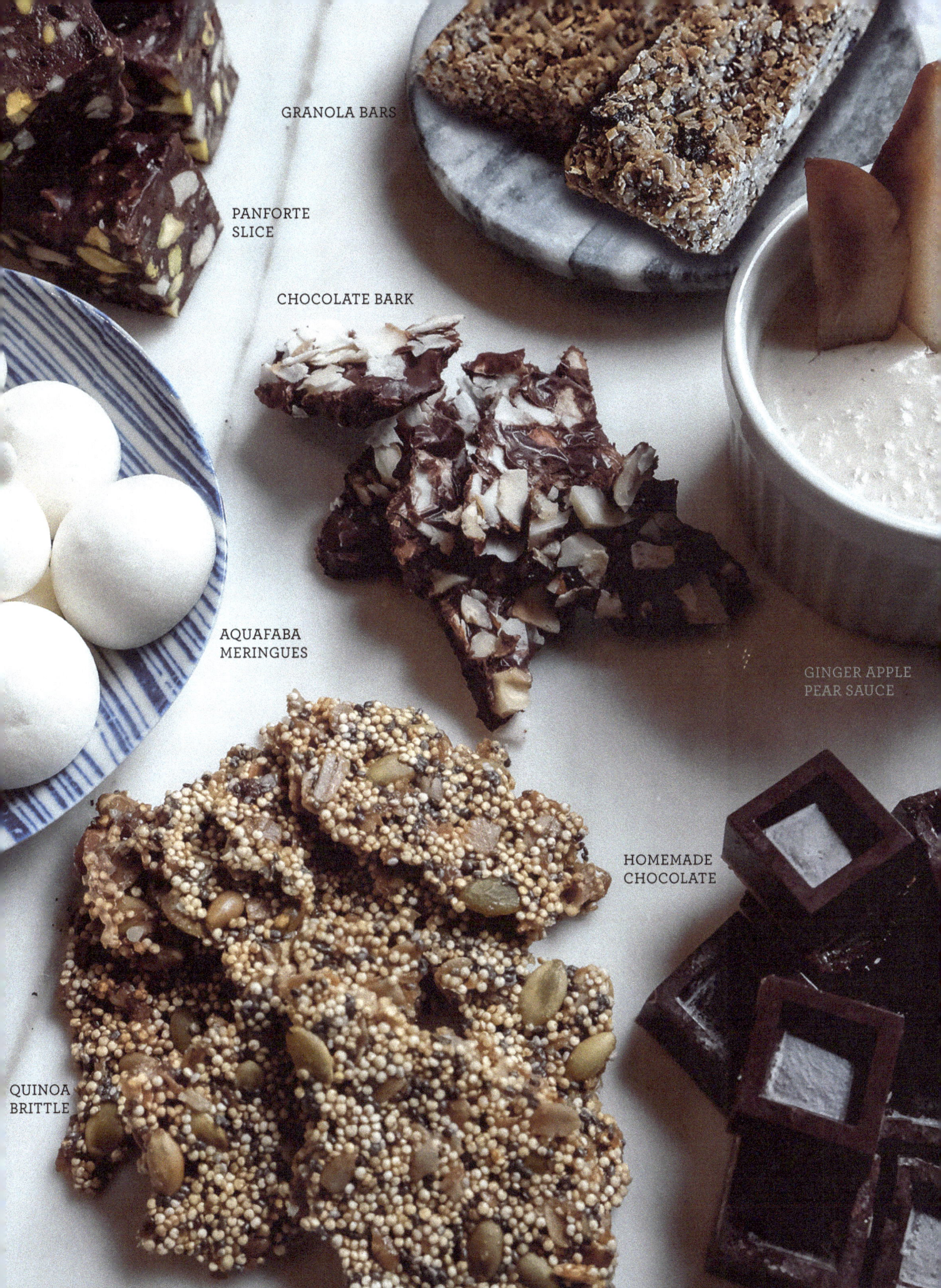

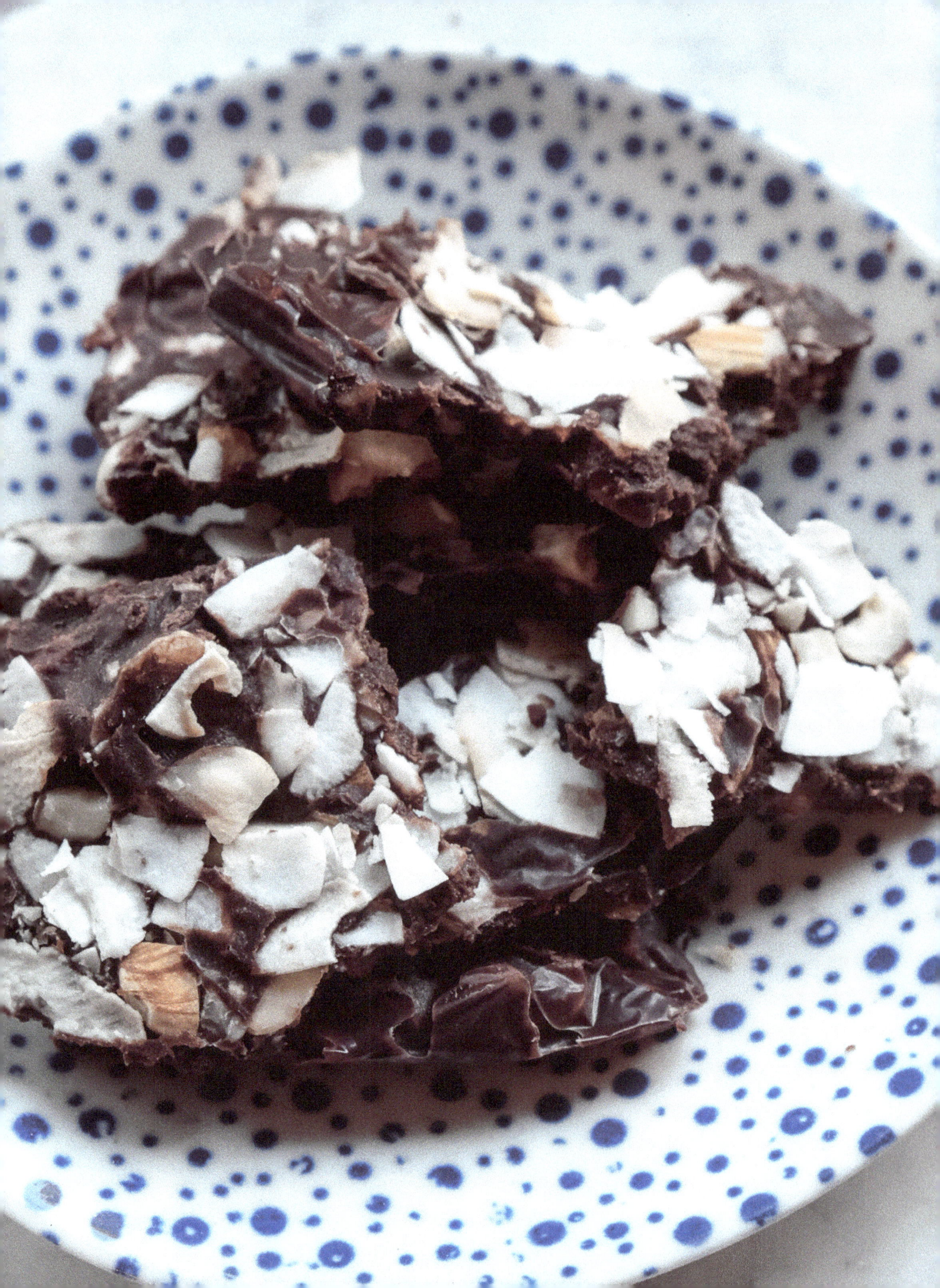

CHOCOLATE BARK

MAKES ABOUT 20 PIECES
KEEP IN AN AIRTIGHT CONTAINER IN THE FREEZER UNTIL READY TO EAT

¼ cup	Almonds, raw
¼ cup	Hazelnuts, raw
¼ cup	Coconut flakes, dried
½ cup	Extra virgin coconut oil
½ cup	Raw cacao powder, sifted
¼ cup	Maple syrup
1 tbsp	Almond butter
Pinch	Sea salt

You need a 23 cm square baking pan or one close to this size.

- Preheat oven to 150°C.
- Line your baking pan with 2 pieces of baking paper, one going each way.
- Line an oven tray with baking paper and add hazelnuts and almonds (keep them separate). Roast for 10 minutes.
- Place roasted hazelnuts in a clean cotton cloth and rub them well until most of the skins fall off. Then roughly chop hazelnuts and almonds.
- On the oven tray, spread out the coconut flakes and roast for 2 minutes (coconut burns quickly).
- In a medium saucepan, melt the coconut oil over low heat.
- Remove from heat and whisk in cacao powder, maple syrup and almond butter.
- Add sea salt to taste and stir in half the chopped almonds and hazelnuts.
- Using a spatula, spoon the chocolate mixture into the prepared pan and smooth out until it is about 1 cm thick.
- Sprinkle on remaining chopped nuts and all the roasted coconut flakes.
- Place into freezer for about 15 minutes, or until frozen.
- Once frozen, remove from freezer and break into pieces.

TIP: This melts fast so when it's removed from freezer, it's time to eat!

VARIATIONS: For a nut-free version, leave out the almond butter, hazelnuts and almonds. You can add toasted pumpkin and sunflower seeds instead of nuts.

Add food-grade mint extract or orange peel for a different flavour.

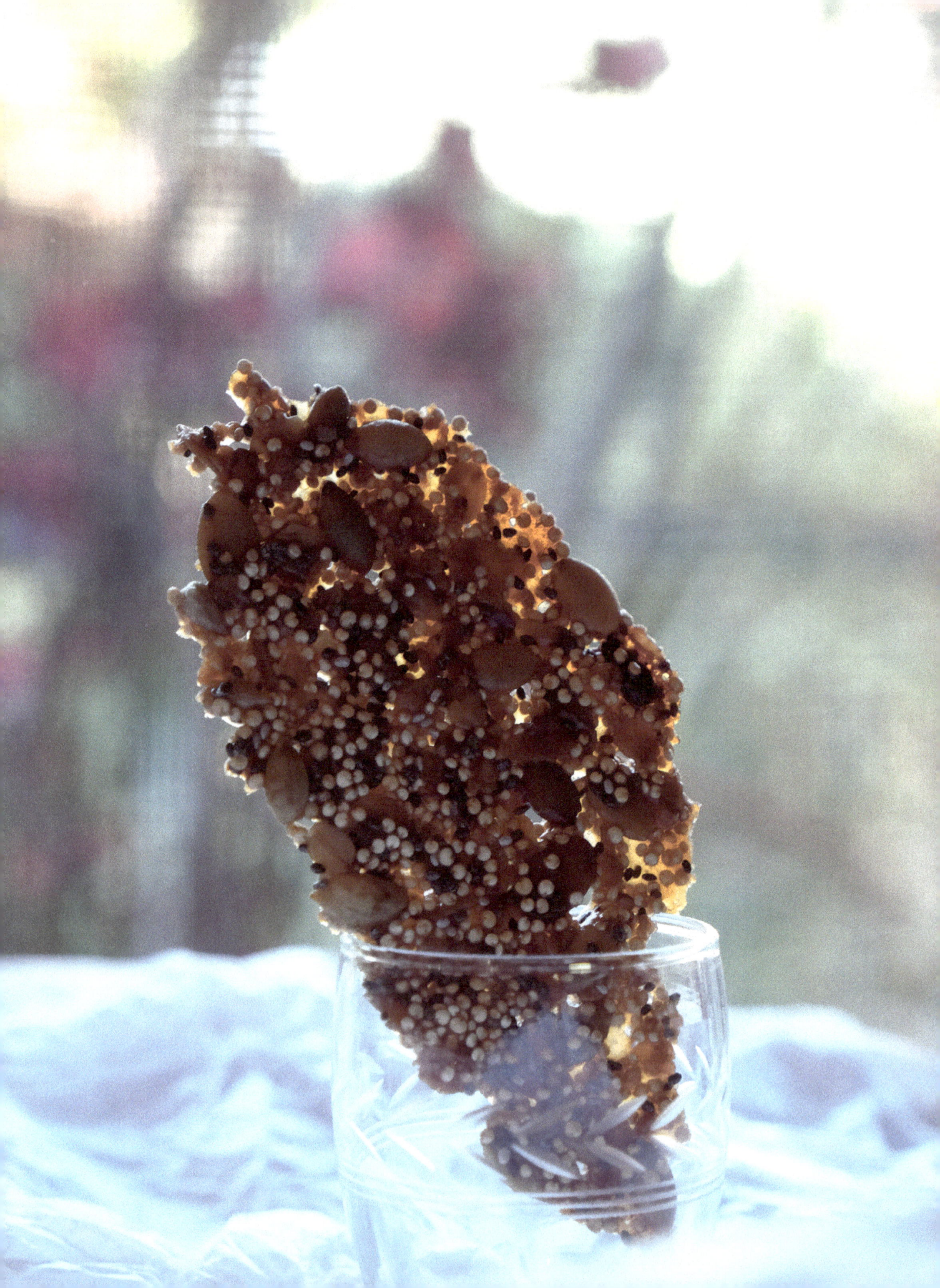

NUT-FREE CRUNCHY QUINOA BRITTLE

KEEP FOR 1 WEEK IN AN AIRTIGHT GLASS JAR OR FOR LONGER IN AIRTIGHT CONTAINER IN FREEZER

½ cup	White quinoa, uncooked
¾ cup	Pumpkin and/or sunflower seeds
¼ cup	Rolled oats
2 tbsp	Chia seeds
2 tbsp	Coconut sugar
Pinch	Sea salt
2 tbsp	Coconut oil (extra virgin for coconut flavour)
½ cup	Maple or coconut syrup

- Preheat oven to 160°C.
- Completely line a baking tray or pan with baking paper.
- In a bowl, mix together quinoa, seeds, oats, chia seeds, coconut sugar and sea salt.
- In a small saucepan, warm the coconut oil and syrup, stirring well over low heat for 2 minutes. Pour this into the bowl of dry ingredients and mix all together.
- Tip onto the lined baking tray and spread the mixture out, getting it as even and flat as possible. (Use a metal spatula.)
- Place in oven and bake for 15 minutes, then turn the tray around to make sure both sides are browned. Bake for 5 minutes more. Keep checking to make sure it does not burn.
- Remove from oven to completely cool before breaking into smaller pieces.

PANFORTE SLICE

MAKES ABOUT 24 PIECES
KEEPS REFRIGERATED IN AN AIRTIGHT CONTAINER FOR A COUPLE OF WEEKS ... IF YOU CAN RESIST

250 g	Almonds, blanched
200 g	Pistachios
150 g	Dried apricots, currants and/or figs
200 g	Dark chocolate
75 g	Candied citrus peel, finely chopped
500 g	Honey, warmed
150 g	Rice flour, sifted
2 tbsp	Raw cacao powder, sifted
½ tsp	Mixed spice
1 tsp	Cinnamon, ground

I use my porcelain baking tray, which measures 27 x 18 cm and is 6 cm deep.

- Preheat oven to 160°C and line a baking dish with baking paper.
- Roast blanched almonds in oven for 10 minutes.
- Chop nuts and dried fruit.
- Melt dark chocolate in a double saucepan.
- Put melted chocolate and chopped nuts, citrus peel and dried fruit in a bowl. Stir in warmed honey until well combined.
- In a separate bowl, combine flour, raw cacao powder, mixed spice and cinnamon then fold through the chocolate mixture.
- Spread the mixture into the prepared pan and bake for 45 minutes or until just set and a little moist.
- Remove from the oven and let cool in the pan before slicing and serving.

PEAR TART

SERVES 6

CRUST

6 tbsp	Chilled coconut oil
1 ¼ cups	Gluten-free flour (I use Orgran gluten-free all-purpose pastry mix)
2 tsp	Organic cane or coconut sugar
¼ tsp	Sea salt
4–6 tbsp	Ice-cold water

FILLING

3	Pears (I use Beurre Bosc pears)
3 tbsp	Currants or raisins
1 tsp	Mixed spice
Pinch	Sea salt
1 cup	Water or pear juice (I use pear juice concentrate for this)
1 tbsp	Kuzu starch

MAKING CRUST

- Coat a pie dish with a little coconut oil.
- In a large mixing bowl, combine gluten-free flour, sugar and sea salt. Mix scoops of the chilled coconut oil gently into your flour (best to use a pastry cutter or fork) until you get a sandy mixture. Leave some of the coconut oil in small pea-sized pieces. Don't overwork the dough.
- Add the ice-cold water a little at a time and mix gently. Add more water as needed (though not more than about 6 tbsp) to form loose dough.
- Knead dough gently with your hands, for up to 1 minute, to form a 1 cm–thick disc. Wrap firmly in plastic wrap and refrigerate for 30 minutes. While it is refrigerating, pre-heat the oven to 190°C. (My oven is electric).
- Remove dough from plastic wrap and place it between 2 large pieces of baking paper. With a rolling pin, gently roll it into shape of your pie pan. (Don't worry if it cracks: once it is placed in the pie pan you can use your fingers to lightly press the dough back together.) Crust should be about 5 mm thick.
- Remove the top layer of baking paper and place the oiled pie dish face-down on the dough. Gently, with the support of the remaining paper, turn the pie dish right-side up. Remove remaining paper.
- Use your hands to gently press the dough into shape, working it up around the sides. (Don't overwork this dough, be gentle.)
- Use a fork to prick all around the bottom to allow steam to escape without the crust bubbling up.
- Place in the pre-heated oven and bake for 20 minutes or until golden brown.
- Remove from oven and place on a cooling rack to completely cool before filling.

COOKING PEARS

- While the crust is cooling, slice pears and place in a saucepan with currants or raisins, mixed spice, sea salt and water or pear juice. Bring to the boil and simmer for 15 minutes or until pears are cooked (add a little more water if necessary).
- Remove pears from saucepan and use remaining liquid in next step.

ASSEMBLING PEAR TART

- Dissolve kuzu in ¼ cup cold water and slowly add, while stirring, to liquid in saucepan. Simmer and stir until transparent. Remove from heat.
- Arrange cooked sliced pears with currants or raisins on crust then pour over kuzu mixture.
- Cool to set. Keep in refrigerator until ready to serve.

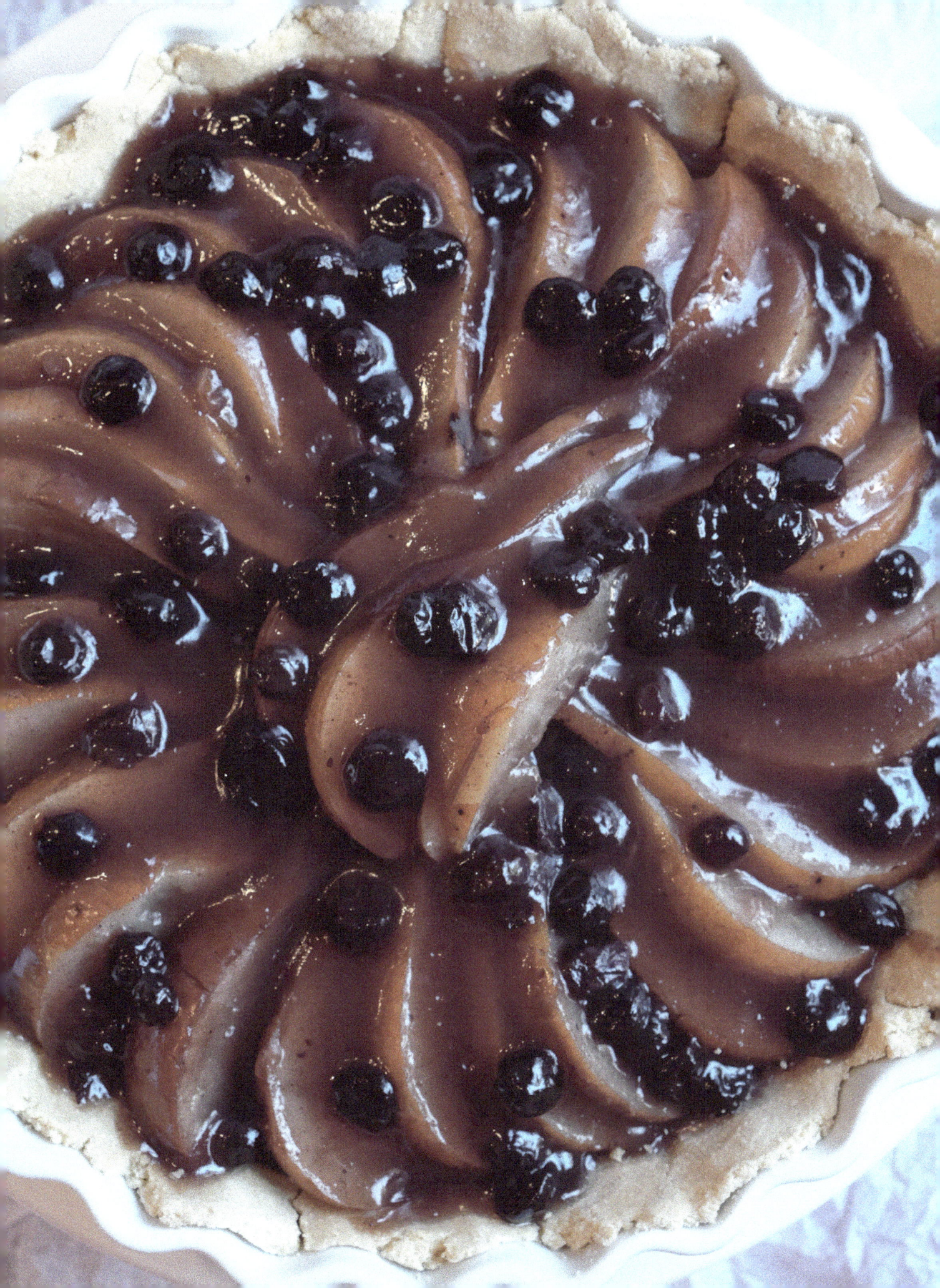

I love chickpeas. Here's an amazing treat to make with the liquid in a tin of cooked chickpeas.

Aquafaba is the name for the viscous water in which legumes, such as chickpeas, have been cooked. Due to its ability to mimic functional properties of egg whites, aquafaba can be used as a direct replacement for egg whites in some recipes. This is so intriguing that I have succumbed to using granulated sugar to make this recipe for special occasions.

AQUAFABA MERINGUES

MAKES ABOUT 30 SMALL MERINGUES
STORE IN AN AIRTIGHT GLASS CONTAINER TO KEEP MERINGUES FROM GETTING SOFT AND STICKY

400 g tin	Chickpeas
½ cup	Granulated sugar (use white sugar if you like your meringues white or coconut sugar for a more golden beige colour)

- Pre-heat oven to 100°C and line an oven tray with baking paper.
- Drain the liquid from the can of chickpeas. You should get about ½ to ¾ cup of liquid.
- Whisk the liquid in a high-speed mixer until stiff peaks form.
- Add the sugar one tbsp at a time. Once the sugar has been incorporated, feel the foam and, if it has any grittiness, keep whisking until the mixture is smooth.
- Dollop 3 cm rounds onto the lined baking tray and bake for 1 ½ hours.
- After cooking time, turn off the oven, crack open the oven door and let the meringues cool to room temperature.

> *I first met Sandra when she was doing the Graduate Diploma of Applied Science in Nutritional & Environmental Medicine at the Graduate School of Integrative Medicine at Swinburne University, when I was the Foundation Head of this post-graduate medical school. What is immediately striking about Sandra is her passion for good, healthy, wholesome food. Sandra's vision encompasses a global perspective, making healthier individuals, communities and a healthier world! Her guiding principle has always been that of Hippocrates – that our 'Food is Medicine'.*
>
> *For over 30 years, Sandra has actively been living her natural food passion – studying, teaching, creating businesses including very successful cooking classes. Years of dedication, research, knowledge and hands-on experience have culminated in Sandra's ultimate, long-anticipated project – My Wholefood Community Cookbook. Sandra's book will inspire your approach to cooking and to becoming a healthier, happier you!*
>
> **Professor Avni Sali AM MBBS PhD FRACS FACS FACNEM, Director – National Institute of Integrative Medicine (Australia), President – International Council of Integrative Medicine (Australia)**

RAW CACAO PROTEIN ENERGY BALLS

MAKES ABOUT 15
KEEPS REFRIGERATED IN A GLASS JAR FOR UP TO 1 WEEK

6	Dried dates or figs
6	Dried apricots (use brown organic apricots)
½ cup	Coconut or rice syrup
½ cup	Tahini (students prefer the taste of hulled tahini)
½ cup	Raw cacao powder
½ cup	Almonds, ground
1 tbsp	Chia seeds
1 tbsp	Miso paste
1 tsp	Cardamom, ground
1 tsp	Cinnamon, ground
1 tbsp	Lemon zest
4–5 tbsp	Lemon juice, to taste
As required	Coconut, ground or almonds, ground (for rolling)

- In a food processor, chop dates or figs and apricots (or finely chop by hand).
- Combine syrup with tahini in a heavy-based saucepan and simmer over a low heat until melted.
- Remove from heat and immediately add into food processor with all ingredients and mix well (or if using your hands then mix in a large bowl).
- Shape into 3 cm diameter balls and set aside for at least 1 hour.
- Roll in ground coconut or ground almonds.

HOMEMADE CHOCOLATE

MAKES 12 SMALL SQUARES, DEPENDING ON MOULD TRAY
BEST KEPT IN FREEZER

¼ cup	Coconut oil (extra virgin for coconut flavour, virgin for neutral flavour)
¼ cup	Raw cacao powder
1½ tbsp	Rice or coconut syrup or honey
½ tsp	Vanilla, ground

Buy a pliable chocolate mould tray.

- Gently melt coconut oil in a saucepan over medium-low heat.
- Stir cocoa powder, sweetener and vanilla into melted oil until well blended.
- Pour mixture into a chocolate mould or pliable tray. Refrigerate until chilled, about 1 hour.

TIPS: This chocolate melts fast so keep chilled until ready to eat.

This recipe is not very sweet so adjust sweeteners to your taste. Note that rice syrup is not as sweet as honey and coconut syrup.

VARIATIONS: Add ground cayenne pepper or chilli oil for a special zing.

Sprinkle on coconut flakes into the mould before pouring in mixture.

Add orange rind to the mixture.

If you like peppermint or any other flavour, buy food-grade flavours to add.

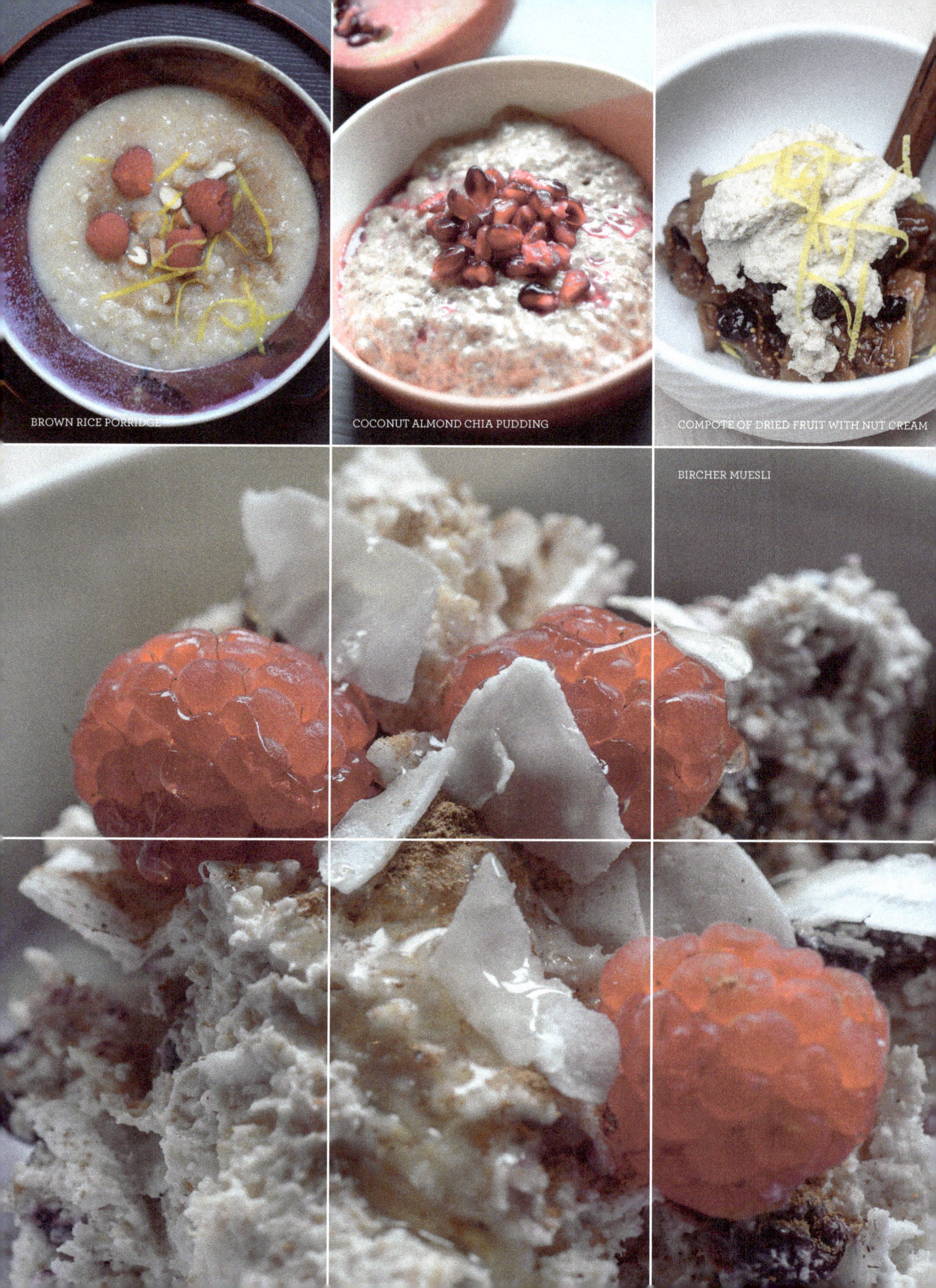

BROWN RICE PORRIDGE

COCONUT ALMOND CHIA PUDDING

COMPOTE OF DRIED FRUIT WITH NUT CREAM

BIRCHER MUESLI

My Favourite Breakfasts

Coconut Chia Almond Pudding.......................... 148

Ted's Oat Granola............................. 148

Bircher Muesli 149

Compote Of Dried Fruits With Nut Cream.................... 149

Brown Rice Porridge 150

Soft Millet Porridge............................. 150

Creamy Quinoa Pudding.................................... 151

COCONUT CHIA ALMOND PUDDING

MAKES ABOUT 2 CUPS
KEEPS REFRIGERATED FOR UP TO 3 DAYS

6 tbsp	Chia seeds
1 cup	Coconut cream
1¼ cups	Almond mylk (see Nut Mylk recipe p.132)
1 tbsp	Vanilla powder (organic tastes best)
2 tbsp	Raw cacao powder
2 tbsp	Rice syrup
Garnish	Pomegranate seeds or berries

- Soak chia seeds overnight in coconut cream and almond mylk.
- Combine all other ingredients in a bowl before adding to chia mix.
- Allow to set for a further 10 minutes.
- Pour into small serving glasses and garnish with pomegranate seeds or berries.

TED'S OAT GRANOLA

STORE IN AN AIRTIGHT GLASS CONTAINER IN A COOL PLACE.
KEEPS BEST FOR 2 WEEKS

¼ cup	Sunflower or safflower oil
¼ cup	Maple syrup
1½ tsp	Pure vanilla extract or powder (organic tastes best)
4 cups	Rolled oats (we like organic or biodynamic rolled oats)
½ cup	Walnuts, chopped
½ cup	Sunflower seeds

Prepare this the night before for your breakfast.

- Preheat oven to 160°C and line a large, shallow oven tray with baking paper.
- Combine liquid ingredients by mixing well in a glass jar or bowl.
- Place rolled oats in a bowl and add liquid ingredients. Mix well to coat.
- Spread mix onto tray and bake for 15 minutes, stirring often, until light golden brown. You can turn tray around too.
- Remove from oven then add chopped walnuts and seeds.
- Return to oven for 5 minutes more.
- Turn off oven and remove mix when golden brown.
- Cool to crisp for about 20 minutes.

I've been making this special mix for my stepfather, Ted, and my mother, Eva, for 15 years. It's part of Ted's daily breakfast.
By the way, they are both in their 90s ... just saying.

BIRCHER MUESLI

SERVES 2–3

1 cup	Rolled oats (organic or biodynamic)
½ cup	Water
½ cup	Yoghurt, organic or biodynamic (I prefer organic coconut yoghurt. It's very creamy and so very delicious)
⅓ cup	Goji berries or currants
⅓ cup	Coconut, shredded or coconut chips (organic is best)
½ tsp	Cinnamon, ground
⅓ cup	Raspberries
	Rice syrup

- In a bowl, mix together oats, water, yoghurt, dried fruit and coconut.
- Cover with a plate and allow to soak overnight in refrigerator.
- Serve for breakfast with cinnamon, raspberries and a drizzle of rice syrup.

VARIATION: Gabrielle prefers to use orange juice instead of water.

COMPOTE OF DRIED FRUITS
With Nut Cream

SERVES 4
ONCE COOLED, THIS KEEPS BEST IN AN AIRTIGHT GLASS CONTAINER IN THE REFRIGERATOR FOR UP TO 1 WEEK

COMPOTE

500 g	Mixed dried fruit (I use organic dried figs and apricots)
½ cup	Currants (organic tastes best)
1	Cinnamon stick
As required	Water
1	Lemon

NUT CREAM
MAKES 1 ½ CUPS

1 cup	Cashews
1 cup	Almonds
2 tbsp	Maple, coconut or rice syrup
1 tsp	Vanilla, ground
½ tsp	Cinnamon, ground
¼–½ cup	Water

COMPOTE

- Cut dried fruit into halves or quarters.
- Place cut dried fruit, currants and cinnamon stick in a saucepan.
- Cover with 5 cm water, bring to the boil and simmer, covered, for 10 minutes.
- While fruit is cooking, zest and juice the lemon.
- Add rind and juice and cook for another 10 minutes.
- Serve warm or cool.

NUT CREAM

- Soak almonds or cashews for at least 1 hour.
- Pulverise the nuts in a high-speed food processor.
- With the machine running, add sweetener, vanilla, cinnamon and enough water to make a creamy consistency.
- This cream usually thickens as it sits; add more water as needed to thin it out.

VARIATION: You can use all almonds, all cashews or both (as I've done).

BROWN RICE PORRIDGE
(Using Pre-Cooked Brown Rice)

SERVES 2-4

2 cups	Brown rice, cooked (see recipe p.82)
1–2 cups	Almond mylk (see Nut Mylk recipe p.132)
¾ cup	Rice syrup
2 tbsp	Lemon or orange zest, to taste
¼ tsp	Pure vanilla extract or powder (organic is best)
Garnish	Nuts, chopped
Garnish	Berries, dried
Garnish	Cinnamon, ground

- Place cooked brown rice in a medium saucepan, stir in almond mylk (use as much as you desire), rice syrup, zest and vanilla.
- Simmer, stirring, for 10 minutes
- Serve with garnishes.

SOFT MILLET PORRIDGE

SERVES 3-4

1 cup	Hulled millet
4 cups	Boiling water
Pinch	Sea salt

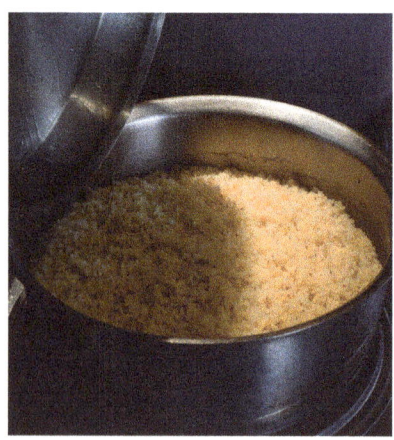

- Wash millet, place in a medium heavy-based saucepan over medium heat and toast for a few minutes until fragrant and beginning to pop, then add boiling water and salt.
- Bring to the boil again, cover and lower heat. Simmer for 30 minutes or until soft enough to serve.

TIP: For a quicker version, place millet in a pan, cover with water and soak overnight. The next morning, place on a low heat and simmer for 15 minutes, adding more water or any nut mylk, as needed.

You can cook millet with raisins or with roasted seeds too.

VARIATIONS: For a savoury porridge, add spring onions, parsley, nori or dulse flakes, and sunflower or chia seeds.

For a sweet porridge, add nut mylk, seeds, a little sweetener, like rice syrup, and compote of dried fruits (see recipe p.149).

CREAMY QUINOA PUDDING

SERVES 3-4

1 cup	Quinoa
2 ½ cups	Almond mylk (see Nut Mylk recipe p.132)
Pinch	Sea salt
1 tbsp	Tahini (I preferred hulled tahini)
2 tbsp	Rice syrup
2 tbsp	Kuzu starch
4 tbsp	Water
1 tbsp	Vanilla, ground
½ tsp	Nutmeg, cinnamon or cardamom, ground

- Wash quinoa well, rinse and drain.
- Place quinoa, almond mylk and salt into a medium heavy-based saucepan and bring to the boil.
- Cover and simmer for 20 minutes.
- Add tahini and rice syrup. Mix well.
- Dissolve kuzu completely in 4 tbsp of water then add to mix in saucepan, stirring constantly until mixture thickens.
- Add vanilla and spice and remove from heat.
- Serve with added berries or seeds.

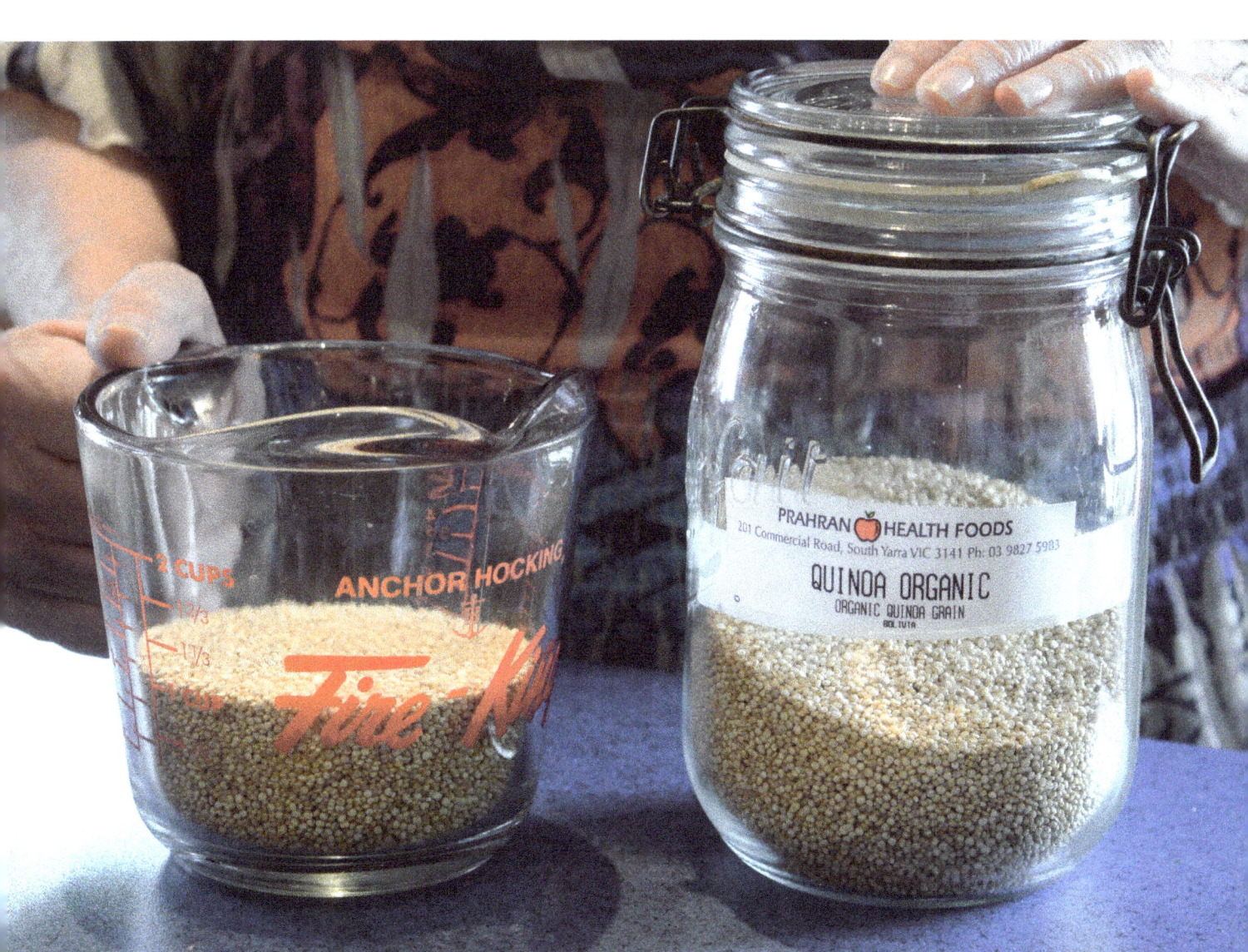

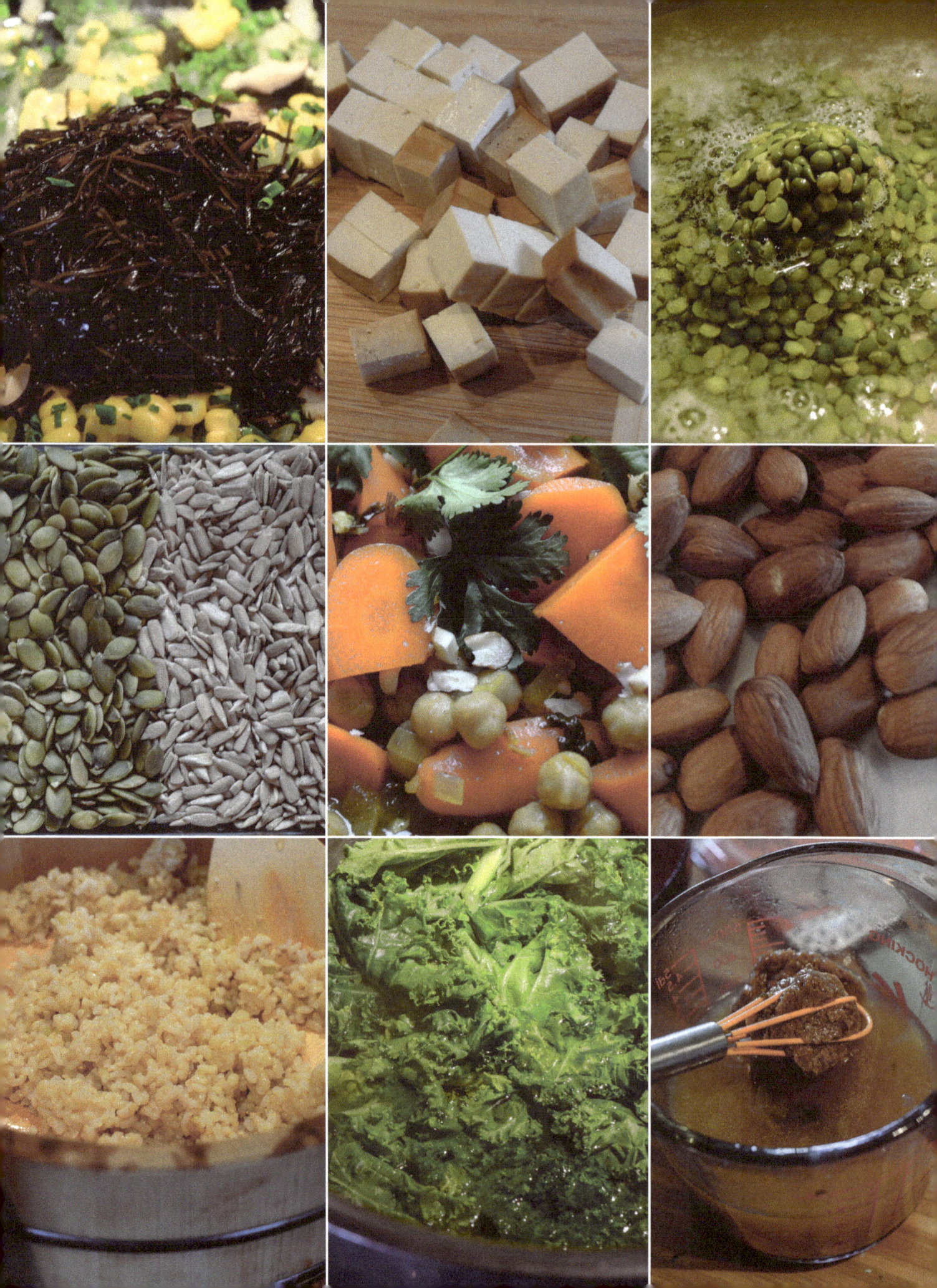

I shared this glossary with so many students as part of the printed class handouts and now I can share it with you.

GLOSSARY

HEALTH BENEFITS OF THE INGREDIENTS

ADZUKI (ADUKI/AZUKI) BEANS

These small, red beans with a nutty flavour originated in China. In Japan they are called the 'king of beans'.

Like many other beans, adzuki are a good source of fibre, protein, magnesium, potassium, iron, zinc, copper, manganese and B vitamins.

Adzuki beans, along with lentils and chickpeas, are a staple of the macrobiotic diet, which calls for the consumption of plenty of fibrous, protein-packed legumes. Macrobiotics consider adzuki to be the most 'yang', or warming, of all beans, and consequently good for imparting strength. Known for their healing properties in traditional Chinese medicine, adzuki beans are said to support kidney, bladder and reproductive function.

ARAME SEA VEGETABLE

A perennial sea vegetable, the arame that I use is grown abundantly on rocks in the Sea of Japan, harvested by hand and naturally sundried during the summer months. Arame is a species of kelp and comes in dark brown strands.

Since its original taste is bitter, steam boiling is used to remove its bitterness. Its mild flavour and firm texture makes it adaptable to many uses.

TIP: *In the Ise-Shima region of Japan, some people use the arame soaking water, which is brown, because it contains iodine, for bathing. It is said to make the skin smoother.*

AQUAFABA

An amazing discovery for me, aquafaba is the name for the viscous water in which legume seeds such as chickpeas have been cooked. Due to its ability to mimic functional properties of egg whites, aquafaba can be used as a direct replacement for egg whites in some recipes.

BEANS

Beans are an inexpensive, low-kilojoule source of protein. They are rich in phytonutrients and antioxidants and are a great source of minerals and B vitamins.

The high-quality carbohydrates, lean protein and soluble fibre of beans help stabilise your body's blood-sugar levels, stave off hunger and give you a steady supply of energy.

Unfortunately, you may be dissuaded from eating beans because of past experiences with gassiness.

The raffinose family of oligosaccharides are complex natural sugars that are largely responsible for the gaseous digestive response to beans and other foods like cabbage and broccoli. Since the human digestive system doesn't have an oligosaccharide enzyme, humans cannot break these sugars down in the digestive tract, and this causes gas.

Although oligosaccharides are present in smaller amounts in a number of fresh vegetables, they are present in large amounts in mature beans, which is why we associate beans with gas. Any bean picked young in the pod and cooked fresh rather than dried will have a much less intense effect. So, while canned or dried pinto, black and kidney beans may trouble you, green beans and other young beans may not.

Green beans, also known as French beans, string beans and snap beans, are the unripe fruit and protective pods of various cultivars of the common bean. They are nutritionally comparable to other pod vegetables, such as snap peas and okra. Green beans are a good source of protein, B vitamins, folate, calcium, iron, magnesium, potassium and fibre. They also contain vitamins A, C and K. In addition, green beans are high in phytonutrients, with an especially wide variety of carotenoids (including lutein and beta-carotene) and flavonoids (including quercetin), which have been shown to have health-supportive antioxidant properties.

Soaking

Soaking dried beans for several hours or overnight drastically reduces the number of oligosaccharides present, which, in turn, reduces flatulent distress during digestion. If you are especially sensitive to beans, you should change the soaking water several times to remove as many oligosaccharides as possible.

Fresh picked beans don't need soaking as their sugars have not yet been converted to long chain carbohydrates that are hard to digest. It's the dried beans that require soaking.

Enzyme supplements

Other ways to reduce the effect of using dried beans are to use kombu sea vegetable when cooking the dried beans or to take over-the-counter supplementation. Kombu sea vegetable, which also contributes minerals, has a special enzyme that helps to break down the complex natural sugars. (A 2 cm piece is plenty for ½ cup of dried beans)

Note: Kombu has been banned only in Australia due to iodine levels, even though many of us are low in iodine, but you can buy it online or you can use wakame, which is freely available but not quite as effective.

You can also buy supplements that contain the enzymes that your digestive system is lacking. These do help to reduce or eliminate flatulence.

Adding digestive spices like ginger, cumin, fennel, caraway, turmeric or asafoetida also helps to make beans more digestible.

Importantly, don't forget to chew your cooked beans and enjoy their flavour! Beans and grains are foods with which digestion starts in the mouth.

According to traditional Chinese medicine, beans strengthen the kidneys, adrenal glands and nervous system, promoting physical growth and development, and provide a 'grounded' kind of energy. While legumes as a category strengthen the kidneys, their colour indicates additional medicinal properties. Green-coloured beans, like mung beans and split peas, also benefit the liver and gall bladder. Red beans, including adzuki and kidney beans, support the heart. Yellow beans like chickpeas and soy beans support the pancreas and stomach. Navy beans, lima and other white beans energise the lungs and colon. Black beans are doubly supportive to the kidneys.

Support your endurance with a bowl of beans, as beans and other legumes (such as peas and lentils) are energising and a comfort food. I recommend organic beans to prevent toxicity from chemically grown and genetically modified crops. If you are buying cooked beans then make sure the tins are BPA free (Bisphenol A). BPA has been recognised as a problematic toxin from the standpoint of the ecosystem and ocean life, and a somewhat controversial toxin with respect to human health.

Storing beans

Uncooked, dry beans should be stored in tightly sealed containers and kept in a cool, dry area. While storage time does not affect nutrient value, beans may require longer cooking times as they age. Cooked beans, if refrigerated, will keep for up to five days in a covered container.

BROWN RICE

It has long been standard practice in macrobiotic cooking to soak brown rice. This was due to anecdotal evidence of its improved digestibility and naturally better flavour.

Now there is scientific proof of the benefits of this practice. A team of Japanese scientists has found that germinating brown rice by soaking it for several hours before it is cooked, enhances its already high nutritional value.

Germinated rice contains much more fibre than conventional brown rice, say the researchers, three times the amount of the essential amino acid lysine, and ten times the amount of gamma-aminobutyric acid (GABA), another amino acid known to improve kidney function.

Various types of analyses on germinated brown rice (GBR) conducted in Japan indicated that during the process of germination, nutrients in the brown rice change drastically. Kayahara et al. (2001) showed that, not only existing nutrients increased but new components are released.

The nutrients which increase significantly include GABA, lysine, vitamin E, dietary fiber, niacin, magnesium, vitamin B1, and vitamin B6 (Kayahara et al. 2001; Kayahara 2001). The other nutrients that increased in GBR were inositols, ferulic acid, phytic acid, tocotrienols, potassium, zinc, g-oryzanol, and prolylendopeptidase inhibitor (Kayahara and Tsukahara 2000).

Further, they found that GBR contains less calories and sugar than that in milled white rice.

Trachoo et al. (2006) found that germination of rice grains increased many nutrients such as vitamin B, reducing sugar, and total protein contents of germinated brown rice were higher than brown rice and white rice.
(See https://www.ncbi.nlm.nih.gov/pmc/articles/PMC3551059)

Wholegrain brown rice contains an ideal balance of minerals, protein and carbohydrates because it retains the outer bran and germ layers of the grain and the vitamins, minerals, fibre and even fatty acids that are housed there.

Brown rice is an excellent source of manganese, and a good source of selenium, phosphorus, copper, magnesium and niacin (vitamin B3). Manganese is a mineral that aids in fatty acid synthesis and protects against free radical damage during energy production. The oil found in the bran of brown rice has also been shown to have special cholesterol-lowering benefits.

Brown rice comes in an array of varieties such as basmati, jasmine and long- and short-grain.

According to traditional Chinese medicine, brown rice strengthens the spleen, nourishes the stomach, strengthens the lungs, relieves irritability and astringes intestines.

Short-grain rice is very starchy and cooks up soft and sticky. It's used in things like sushi, paella and risotto.

Long-grain rice contains less starch so the cooked grains are drier and more separate. It's often used in pilafs or dishes with a lot of sauce.

I recommend organic or, even better, biodynamic brown rice.

Storing cooked rice

When it comes to storing cooked rice, store it in the fridge for two days – no more. Do not leave cooked rice on the kitchen bench for extended periods as rice can foster bacteria. Its high levels of carbohydrate make it a breeding ground for nasty bugs, so as soon as your cooked rice reaches room temperature, transfer it to an airtight container and store it in the fridge.

It is best to store uncooked brown rice in the freezer because it contains a very small amount of fat and will go rancid if left too long on the shelf. If you don't have room in your freezer, at least store your rice in the fridge.

BROWN RICE VINEGAR

I use Japanese organic brown rice vinegar, a naturally fermented seasoning, which is aged for one year using traditional methods. Made from organic brown rice, it is fermented in 100-year-old earthenware vats that are buried in the ground.

Brown rice vinegar preserves the nutrients and freshness of salad vegetables and is essential for making sushi rice, pickles and dressings. This vinegar is rich in minerals and organic acids that stimulate metabolism and support a healthy blood condition. Even though it is generally used as cooking vinegar, brown rice vinegar is also popularly considered a healthy drink that is good for digestion. You can drink it with honey.

BIODYNAMIC FOOD

Biodynamics is a holistic, ecological and ethical approach to farming, gardening, food and nutrition. Biodynamics was first developed in the early 1920s based on the spiritual insights and practical suggestions of the Austrian writer, educator and social activist Dr Rudolf Steiner (1861–1925), whose philosophy is called 'anthroposophy'.

While similar to organic farming, biodynamic farming principles have a greater focus on astrological cycles and the idea of the farm as a single 'organism'. Biodynamic farmers use unique soil, plant and compost preparations that, when done successfully, create a humus-rich, well-structured soil that is ideal for the growth of healthy, vibrant plants. Under the respectful work of the farmer, the plant grows in tune with nature and the pure influence of the sun and cosmos.

CACAO – RAW, ORGANIC

Used as a food, a medicine and a currency, cacao has been cultivated throughout Mexico, Central America and South America since the Early Formative Period (1900–900 BC). Cacao was so highly valued that the ancient native peoples celebrated it and used it in rituals and everyday life, immortalising its place in their society through oral history, stonework and pottery. Cacao is part of the Mayan Creation Myth, and is believed to be of divine origin. Theobroma means 'food of the gods' and cacao, or Theobroma cacao, is the source of original, natural chocolate. It comes from seeds of the fruit of the cacao tree. Raw cacao powder is made by cold-pressing unroasted beans. The process keeps the living enzymes in the cocoa and removes the fat.

This moderately addictive plant-derived substance contains amazingly powerful nutrients. Raw cacao powder has more than 300 phytochemicals and nearly four times the antioxidant power of regular dark chocolate, and contains protein, calcium, carotene, thiamine, riboflavin, magnesium, and sulfur.

There are studies showing its beneficial effect on cardiovascular system, including lowering blood pressure, lipid levels and insulin resistance. Fringe benefits of cacao are that it releases into the brain chemicals that improve cognitive function and mood. It's no wonder the Spanish called it 'black gold'.

Fun fact: The Aztecs gave cacao the name *yollotl eztli*, meaning 'heart blood'. They may have understood even then the heart-benefiting aspects of eating cacao, which we now know is a boost for the cardiovascular system.

Note: Too much raw cacao is not healthy. Cacao is an extremely addictive substance. Much like coffee, raw cacao acts as a stimulant, so remember that cacao is still a treat.

Store organic raw cacao in an airtight container in a dark, cool, dry place.

CHIA SEEDS

It is believed chia seeds were first grown and harvested by the Aztecs during the pre-Columbian era. This plant, Salvia hispanica, is an annual herb and a member of the mint family. The ancient civilisation believed that the chia seed from this plant provided supernatural powers. In Mayan, chia means 'strength'. Aside from eating it, the Aztecs used the chia seed for many things: it was used in medicine, ground into flour, mixed as an ingredient in drinks, and pressed for oil. It was useful in that it could be stored for relatively long periods of time (perfect for travelling). In addition to these practical uses, the chia seed was sacred to the Aztecs, who used it as a sacrifice in religious ceremonies.

Chia seeds are rich in fibre, omega-3 fats, protein, vitamins and minerals. Chia seeds are considered to be an unprocessed wholegrain food. Chia seeds are gluten free and best are organic, non-GMO.

Chia seeds form a sort of gel when mixed with liquid, so can be substituted for eggs or used as a soup thickener and can also be included in all kinds of baked goods for some added energy.

CRUCIFEROUS VEGETABLES

Vegetables of the family Brassicaceae (also called Cruciferae) are widely cultivated, with many genera, species and cultivars.

Included in this group of vegetables are: rocket, bok choy, broccoli, brussels sprouts, cabbage, cauliflower, Chinese broccoli, Chinese cabbage, collard greens, daikon, horseradish, kale, kohlrabi, mizuna, mustard plants, pak choy, radishes (red and daikon), rutabaga, tatsoi, turnips, wasabi and watercress.

Cruciferous vegetables are high in antioxidants, which help reduce oxidative stress, and rich in nutrients, including carotenoids (beta-carotene, lutein, zeaxanthin), vitamins (C, E and K) folate, protein, iron, chlorophyll, omega-3 fatty acids, calcium and magnesium.

Cruciferous vegetables are anti-inflammatory and health agencies recommend that we eat several servings per week.

DAIKON RADISH

Daikon is a mildly flavoured, low-calorie, nutritious winter radish that is characterised by fast-growing leaves and a long, white root. It is a member of the highly nutritious Brassica family, meaning it's a cousin to cabbage and other cruciferous vegetables.

Daikon has long been considered a superfood in many Asian cultures because of its ability to re-balance the digestive system, boost the immune system and gently cleanse the body.

According to traditional Chinese medicine, daikon is used for indigestion, such as bloating and sluggish bowel movements. Daikon can be cooked in soups and used raw in salads, pickled, stir-fried and grated to aid in the digestion of oily food. (It is served with dipping sauce with Japanese tempura.)

As with all varieties of radish, daikon radishes are a great snack with a high nutritional content that includes vitamins A, C, E and B6, potassium, magnesium, calcium, iron and fibre.

For extra flavour and nutrition, use the whole plant by adding the fresh radish tops to salads.

FERMENTED FOODS AND PICKLES

The earliest record of fermentation dates back as far as 6000 BC in the Middle East, and nearly every civilisation since has at least one fermented food in its culinary heritage. From Korean kimchi and Indian chutneys to sauerkraut, yogurt and cheese, global cultures have crafted unique flavours and traditions around fermentation.

Links between fermented foods and health can be traced as far back as ancient Rome and China, and remain an area of great interest for researchers in modern times.

Natural pickling and fermentation are the most unique, traditional forms of food preservation that enhance the quality of the foods. Fermentation is an external, pre-digestion process that converts complex nutrients to simpler ones. Common fermented foods and beverages include sourdough, vinegar and wine. Pickling is a type of controlled fermentation that uses salt. Examples of pickled products are miso, sauerkraut and olives.

When pickled and fermented foods, which are sources of probiotics, are combined with prebiotics, they help create the healthiest environment for gut microbes to flourish.

For healthy digestion, we need both prebiotics and probiotics. However, they play different roles.

Probiotics: These are live bacteria found in certain foods (naturally found in cultured or fermented foods such as yoghurt, buttermilk, aged cheese, sauerkraut, kimchi, sourdough bread, miso, tempeh and kombucha) or supplements. They can provide numerous health benefits.

Prebiotics: These substances come from types of carbohydrates (mostly fibre) that humans can't digest. The beneficial bacteria in your gut eat this fibre. Prebiotics such as fructooligosaccharides (FOS) and galactooligosaccharides (GOS) are naturally found in many plant based foods.

According to macrobiotics, the basis of a healthy plant-based diet is grains, beans, vegetables and fruits, all prebiotics. The most important probiotics for this way of eating are miso (grain and bean), sauerkraut (vegetable) and umeboshi plum (fruit).

Non-commercially made pickles help protect the body against infections, stimulate the immune system, improve the digestion process, and act as antioxidants. In addition, they also facilitate the synthesis of certain vitamins, such as vitamins C and B.

FLAXEGGS

Flaxeggs are a great baking alternative for vegans and for those who have allergies and must follow an egg-free diet.

Flaxegg (egg substitute) Recipe
- 1 tbsp ground flaxseeds
- 3 tbsp water (to replace 1 egg)

Mix ground flaxseeds with water and let set for 10 minutes before adding to recipe.

GINGER

The root, or rhizome, of the plant Zingiber officinale has been a popular spice and herbal medicine for thousands of years. It has a long history of use in Asian, Indian and Arabic herbal traditions. In China, for example, ginger has been used to help digestion and treat stomach upset, diarrhoea and nausea for more than 2000 years. Ginger has also been used to help treat arthritis, colic and heart conditions.

Today, healthcare professionals may recommend ginger to help prevent or treat nausea and vomiting from motion sickness, pregnancy and cancer chemotherapy. Ginger may help treat the common cold, flu-like symptoms, headaches, painful menstrual periods, mild stomach upset and osteoarthritis.

Ginger is botanically related to turmeric and both have both been used for centuries as spices in cooking and as medicinal herbs.

KALE

This super green is packed to the max with nutrition. It is a member of the cabbage family (brassica oleracea) and therefore related to vegetables like cabbage, broccoli, cauliflower, collard greens and brussels sprouts.

It seems that, in Australia, kale has become popular only in the last few years. I remember going to the market with my mother when I was very young and seeing kale used to decorate the produce displays, as kale looked green for a long time. Now people are eating kale in salads, soups, smoothies and juices.

However, kale is not a new food discovery. Kale and other cabbages have been cultivated for over 2000 years. Though it grows in warm climates, it's happiest in colder climates, such as north Europe, where for centuries its high vitamin content made it especially popular. Until the end of the fifteenth century, kale was one of the most common green vegetables in Europe.

KOMBU

Kombu, a deep-sea kelp, is a sea vegetable of the Laminaria family, of which there are more than ten species. Highly valued in Japan for its medicinal value as well as culinary use, it was prescribed by folk healers for hypertension. High in many essential minerals vitamins, and trace elements, kombu also contains the amino acid glutamine, a naturally sweet flavour enhancer.

Kombu greatly increases the nutritional value of all food prepared with it, as it is considered the most completely mineralised food.

It is widely used in soup stock and dashi broth as a flavour enhancer, and it can be added to beans or root vegetables for improved flavour and a softer texture.

Make sure you buy kombu that grows wild and is gathered by hand from the sea. (Lesser grades of commercial kombu are cultivated artificially or simply gathered from the beach after they wash ashore. Many are sprayed with chemically produced and toxic monosodium glutamate.)

FYI: The white powder on the surface of kombu is the substance for its main flavour; therefore, kombu should not be washed but wiped with a clean cloth.

FYI: Use sparingly, if at all, during pregnancy and avoid in cases of diarrhoea.

Note: Kombu has been banned only in Australia due to iodine levels even though many of us are low in iodine, but you can buy it online or you can use wakame, which is freely available but not quite as effective.

KUKICHA TWIG TEA

My favourite tea is Japanese roasted Kukicha tea, which I have served for the past 30 years as a welcoming tea for all my students and clients. (see photo back cover)

- Kukicha is Japanese for twig tea as it is made from stems and branches that are separated from the Camellia sinensis plant during the refining process that makes Sencha (green tea).
- Kukicha is low in stimulants. The stems and branches are roasted in cast-iron cauldrons to lessen bitterness and to decrease tannin.
- Favoured among macrobiotics as it contains almost no caffeine.

It is best to simmer Kukicha in a heat-resistant glass pot or saucepan for up to 20 minutes to release deep, full bodied flavour and to make it a more warming drink. For a more cooling beverage, it is steeped. During hot summer, it is best enjoyed as cold tea.

Twig tea does not overly stimulate and therefore can be consumed many times per day.

KUZU (KUDZU)

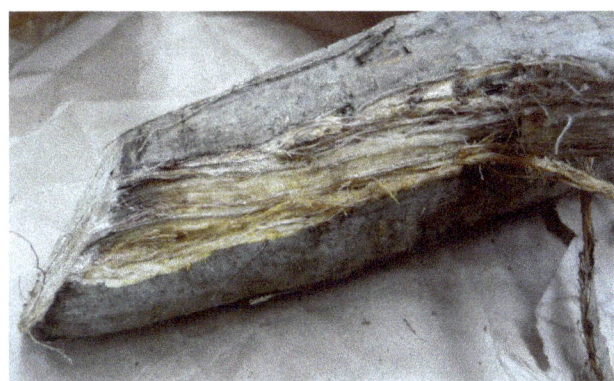

Kuzu root

Kuzu is a starch that is made from the vine plant and root of a tree grown in the high mountains of Japan. It is used in food (especially the root) and in Oriental medicine as a herbal beverage, which is considered to be effective for reducing fevers, alleviating stiff muscles and treating colds, intestinal trouble, high blood pressure, blood infections, food poisoning, hangovers and fatigue.

Kuzu starch is a superior thickener that does not separate after cooking and is used to thicken soups, sauces and dressings.

My favourite macrobiotic home remedies using kuzu:

Stomach-Settling Kuzu Cream

Makes 1 cup

This rejuvenating tonic is most effective when taken about one hour before meals (preferably in the morning when the stomach is empty). This recipe makes a thick, pudding-like cream. If you'd prefer to make a thinner drink, reduce the amount of kuzu to one rounded teaspoon.

- 1½ tablespoons kuzu starch
- 1 umeboshi plum, pitted and minced, or 1 teaspoon umeboshi paste
- ¼–½ teaspoon fresh ginger juice (finely grate ginger root and squeeze to extract juice)
- ½–1 teaspoon shoyu (optional)

In a small enamel or non-metallic saucepan, thoroughly dissolve kuzu starch in 1 cup cold water.

Add umeboshi and bring to a simmer over medium heat, stirring frequently. As soon as the mixture begins to bubble around the edges, stir constantly until kuzu thickens and becomes translucent.

Gently simmer 1 to 2 minutes, then remove from heat. Add ginger juice and, if desired, shoyu to taste.

Apple–Kuzu Drink

Serves 1

For a quick pick-me-up or for treating small children, good-tasting kuzu beverages are ideal. In his book, *Macrobiotic Home Remedies*, macrobiotic teacher Michio Kushi recommends Apple–kuzu drink for constipation, fever and to stimulate appetite. The drink's soothing effect is also used to calm down hyperactive children. When making this tonic for young children, replace ½ cup of the apple juice with water.

- 1 cup apple juice
- small pinch sea salt (optional)
- 1 rounded teaspoon kuzu (crush chunks with back of spoon before measuring)
- 1–2 tablespoons water for dissolving kuzu

Heat the apple juice and salt in a small saucepan over medium heat until it just begins to bubble around the edges. Remove from heat.

Thoroughly dissolve the kuzu in water, add it to the juice while stirring, and then return the pot to the burner. Stir constantly until kuzu thickens and becomes translucent.

Simmer a minute more, and then remove from heat. Allow to cool for a few minutes before serving.

LENTILS

The lentil plant (Lens culinaris) is an edible pulse that originates from Asia and North Africa and is one of our oldest sources of food. A cousin to the pea and a rich provider of protein and carbohydrates, the lentil is an easy-to-digest, good source of calcium, phosphorus, iron and B vitamins – making it an important diet staple the world over. To make a complete protein, add lentils to wholegrains, nuts and seeds. (I like adding tahini.)

Cooking lentils

Before cooking lentils, rinse in cold water, pick over to remove debris or shrivelled lentils and then drain. Wait to add salt or any acidic ingredients until the lentils are done cooking. These ingredients can cause the lentils to stay crunchy even when fully cooked. If you stir in salt while the lentils are still warm, they will absorb just enough to taste fully seasoned.

Lentils do not require it but they can be soaked in order to reduce cooking time by about half.

Storing lentils

Keep lentils in an airtight container in a cool, dry place. Although lentils can be kept indefinitely, they are best enjoyed within one year of purchase.

Cooked lentils may be refrigerated for up to one week in a sealed container.

MACROBIOTICS

Macrobiotics – meaning a large or great life – is a philosophy based on quality lifestyle that includes a simple balanced diet of traditional foods, such as wholegrains, beans and locally grown vegetables, as primary sources of food energy and nutrition. Together with the application of Zen Buddhist and Oriental philosophy and medicine, this universal way of life embraces awareness of such things as breathing, exercise, relationships, customs, cultures, ideas and consciousness. It is more than simply a diet.

According to the Merriam-Webster dictionary, macrobiotics is 'of, relating to, or being a diet based on the Chinese cosmological principles of yin and yang that consists of whole cereals and grains supplemented especially with beans and vegetables'.

I started my focus on foods as medicines by direct learning and experience. I was inspired many years ago when I had the privilege of attending classes with Michio Kushi, Herman and Cornelia Aihara (Vega Study Center), David and Cynthia Briscoe (Macrobiotic America) and Annemarie Colbin (Natural Gourmet Institute. NYC). All wise, sincere and knowledgeable human beings dedicated to the wellbeing of all.

MILLET

Millet is the generic name given to more than 6000 species of wild annual grasses found throughout the world. Millet in its various species sustains more than one-third of the world's population.

China, India and Niger are the world's largest growers of millet today. The Hunza people living in the remote Himalayan foothills enjoy millet as their staple grain; they are known for their extraordinary health and longevity.

Millet seed is used as birdseed. Its hard, indigestible hull must be removed before it can be used for human consumption (use hulled millet for cooking). Hulling does not affect the nutrient value as the germ stays intact through this process. Though technically a seed, millet is categorised as a grain from a culinary perspective.

According to traditional Chinese medicine, millet is cooling in nature and is used to stop vomiting, relieve diarrhoea, promote urination, soothe morning sickness, and tone the stomach and intestines. Hulled millet is highly nutritious, gluten-free and is not acid-forming, so it is soothing and easy to digest.

It is suitable for porridge, casseroles, stuffing, side dishes, soups and gluten-free recipes. The consistency can be anywhere from creamy to fluffy, depending on how it is cooked.

Since it is a small grain, millet does not require soaking but pan-toasting will give it a nuttier taste.

MIRIN

Known as sweet sake, mirin is a delicious sweet natural cooking wine containing amino acids, vitamins and enzymes and is used in all types of cooking. For my recipes, I use traditionally made mirin, made from sweet brown rice, rice koji and sea salt.

Prior to the 16th century, sweet sake was made from refined sake and steamed rice koji. The end product, called renshu, had very low alcohol content and a short shelf life. Eventually mirin was created by using distilled spirits with higher alcohol content, producing a precious liquid that was sweeter and longer lasting. Initially, mirin was widely drunk as sweet alcohol but by the 17th century it had caught on as a useful flavouring ingredient in eastern Japan. By the middle of the 19th century, no Japanese household was without it.

Today mirin is known and used throughout the world for its unique sweet flavour.

MISO

Miso means 'fermented beans' in Japanese. A traditional and indispensable ingredient in Japanese and Chinese diets, miso paste is made from fermented soybeans and grains and contains millions of beneficial bacteria that help maintain good gut health. Miso is rich in essential minerals and a good source of various B vitamins, vitamins E and K and folic acid. In Japan, people begin their day with a bowl of miso soup, which is believed to stimulate digestion and energise the body.

The protein-rich paste is highly popular as it provides an instant flavour foundation. It adds the fifth taste, known as umami, to all sorts of dishes including soups and broths, salad dressings, vegetables, stews, glazes and marinades.

The history of miso began in the 6th century AD. In the beginning, miso was a precious, expensive product and was reserved for noblemen. It was often used to pay wages for high-ranking officers. Miso soup was first created in the 12th century by mashing miso grains into hot water. By the 14th century, miso had become available to the common people. In the 15th century, miso pastes were being developed in the home, and it is from this practice that the many kinds of miso developed.

The flavour, texture, colour and degree of saltiness of miso depend on where it is produced (which is why different varieties are associated with different regions), how long it ferments for, if it is pasteurised and which ingredients are used. The darker the miso, the stronger the flavour. Light miso is sweeter as it is the least fermented and made from white rice. The more expensive, traditionally made miso (which I recommend in my recipes) is aged for 18 months to two years and is superior to commercial miso, which has been chemically induced and has shorter fermentation periods. Unpasteurised organic miso is aged for at least two years and contains more enzymes and live bacteria than pasteurised miso.

These are my favourite traditional miso pastes supplied by Spiral Foods (Australia)

Kome miso: Made from soybeans and white rice (non-GMO, gluten-free)

Hatcho miso: Made from pure soybeans (non-GMO, gluten-free, unpasteurised, organic)

Genmai miso: Made from soybeans and brown rice (non-GMO, gluten-free, unpasteurised, organic)

Mugi miso: Made from soybeans and barley (non-GMO, unpasteurised, organic)

Shiro miso: Made from soybeans and white rice and fermented quickly (non-GMO, gluten-free, organic)

Miso has, for centuries, been aged in cedar kegs, and my favourite miso pastes (from Spiral Food and Muso International, Japan) continue to be processed in this same method. Traditionally aged miso uses only the natural ambient temperature, which makes a stronger, more healthful miso, and it has no artificial additives.

Shiro miso, a light miso, has a smooth, creamy texture and a flavour that's mild, slightly tart and a little sweet. According to oriental medicine, it's cooling and therefore great to use in soups, sauces, dips, spreads and dressings in warmer seasons and climates.

The dark miso pastes are more warming to the body and therefore more appropriate for colder seasons and climates.

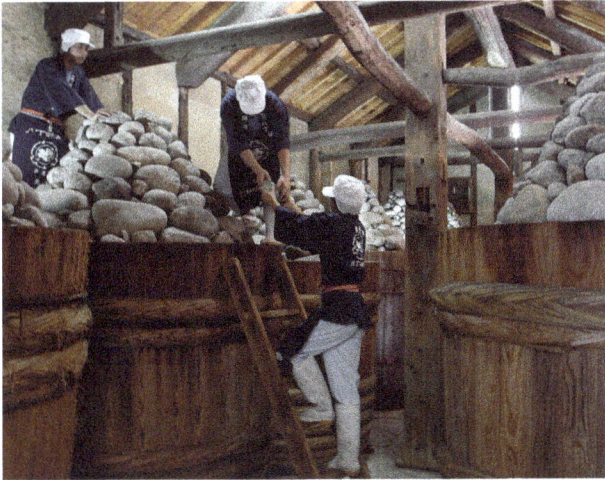

Fermenting miso — Photo: Muso International, Japan

Dark miso provides a great flavour for cooked beans, stews, sauces and soup of all varieties, not just miso soup. To protect its taste, colour, and texture, I recommend refrigerating miso pastes after opening, preferably in a tightly sealed glass jar. When properly stored in the refrigerator, miso can last for many years, in part due to its high concentration of salt.

In general, 1 teaspoon of dark miso is approximately equivalent to 1½ to 2 teaspoons of light miso, which, in turn, is equivalent to about an 1/8 teaspoon of salt.

NOODLES

Noodles have been a staple food in many parts of the world for at least 2000 years. The Chinese, Arabs and Italians have all laid claim to creating the first noodle but the earliest record appears in a book written in China between 25 and 220 AD. Additionally, in 2005, some 4000-year-old noodles – the oldest noodles ever found – were discovered inside an overturned sealed bowl buried under three metres of sediment in Qinghai, in northwest China. Noodles are quick to prepare, easy to chew and enjoyed by young and old. There are many varieties to choose from, as they can be made from wheat, rice, buckwheat and starches derived from pulses, potato and sweet potato.

NORI SEA VEGETABLE

Nori is commonly used as a wrap for sushi and onigiri. It is also a tasty garnish or flavouring in noodle preparations and soups. It is most typically toasted prior to consumption (known as yaki-nori or sushi nori) and has a subtly sweet and complex umami flavour. Natural nori has a deep, rich purple-black colour and a fragrant aroma.

As for nutrition, two 21 cm x 19 cm sheets of nori provide almost half the daily minimum requirements of vitamin A, and also considerable amounts of vitamins B1 and B2.

ORGANIC FOOD

Organic food is the product of a farming system which avoids the use of man-made fertilisers, pesticides, growth regulators and livestock feed additives. Irradiation and the use of genetically modified organisms (GMOs) or products produced from or by GMOs are generally prohibited by organic legislation. Organic products may be certified by voluntary organisations or government bodies.

OYSTER MUSHROOMS

First cultivated in Germany as a subsistence measure during World War I and now grown commercially around the world for food, oyster mushrooms are fleshy, gilled mushrooms that grow in a shelf-like fashion on wood. They are a good food source and are promising medicinally. Oyster mushrooms are native to both deciduous hardwood and conifer tree species and are found in forestlands around the world.

These mushrooms are a great source of protein, copper, potassium, zinc, selenium and B vitamins. Mushrooms are also a great source of fibre and are low in both saturated and unsaturated fat.

Oyster mushrooms show activity against cancer and high cholesterol as well as in anti-tumour, immune response, anti-inflammatory, antiviral and antibiotic areas.

QUINOA

Quinoa, pronounced 'keen-wa', comes from the high plains of the Andes Mountains in South America, where it is known as 'the mother grain' for its life-giving properties. It was one of the staple foods, along with corn and potatoes, of the ancient South American civilisations. For over 5000 years, this wholegrain (actually a pseudo-grain, because it's cooked like grain but is the seed of a beet relative) has been a staple of local diets. Bolivia and Peru account for 90 per cent of world quinoa production today. Quinoa has in the past decade become a popular food and we treat the seeds as we would a grain, preparing and eating them in much the same way. The quinoa plant is actually a relative of beets, spinach and Swiss chard.

Available in light brown, red and even black varieties and now referred to as a 'supergrain', quinoa is easy to digest and a great alternative for people with wheat, gluten and corn allergies.

Quinoa is high in magnesium, is a good source of manganese, iron, copper, phosphorous, vitamin B2 and other essential minerals, and has the highest protein content of any grain. It is especially high in lysine, an amino acid that is typically low in other grains. Quinoa's protein is complete, containing all nine essential amino acids – a rarity in the plant kingdom.

SEA SALT

Humanity has been eating unrefined salt for thousands of years. The word salary comes from the same root as the word salt because salt was such a valuable commodity it was used for currency. Salt is a mineral that has been used worldwide since antiquity as a flavouring, preservative, medicine and sacred offering. It is composed mainly of sodium chloride, which is part of the class of ionic salts. In its natural form, salt is called rock salt or halite. In its edible form, it can be purchased as sea, table, kosher and iodised salt. The main differences between sea salt and table salt are in their tastes, texture and processing.

FYI: Commercial salts are bleached and often have additives such as aluminium compounds to prevent caking.

Organic unrefined sea salt comes from evaporated sea water and is minimally processed, so it may retain trace minerals. The minerals sea salt contains depend on the body of water from which it is evaporated. This may promote a different taste or colour in the salt. Unrefined sea salt is often greyish-white, and sometimes pink or orange. Sea salt can be fine or coarse in texture and comes as crystals and flakes. Flaked sea salt dissolves faster than other types of salt.

I use unrefined and refined grey and white sea salt. Choose a good organic, additive-free sea salt by buying only small quantities and tasting a variety to decide which you prefer. Just remember not to eat too much – the recommended daily intake for sodium that has been set for Australian adults is 1600 mg (equivalent to about four grams of salt).

Good quality, unrefined sea salt is said to have an alkalinising effect on the body and is an extremely yang food in Chinese medical terminology.

SHIITAKE MUSHROOMS

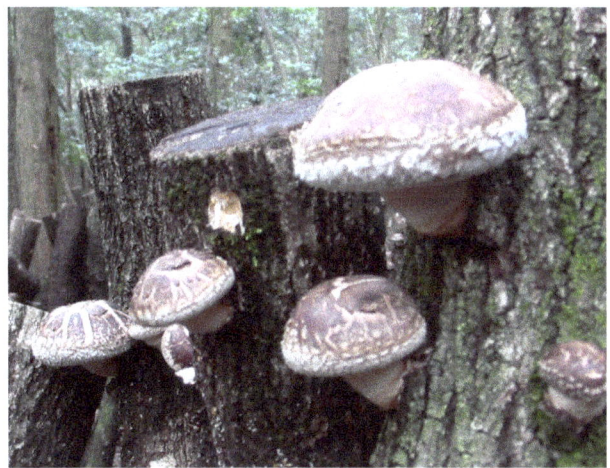

Growing shiitake by traditional methods in Japan   Photo: Muso International Japan

Known as the 'elixir of life' since ancient times, the meaty and flavourful shiitake mushroom is widely referred to as a medicinal mushroom due to its long history of medical use, particularly in oriental medicine traditions. Shiitake mushrooms have traditionally been used as an anti-tumour, antifungal, antiviral and anti-arthritic medicinal food.

As a parasite on a tree, shiitake mushrooms contain strong compounds that have been studied and shown to reduce inflammation, improve the immune system and lower cholesterol.

Shiitake mushrooms are rich in B vitamins and concentrated in minerals, being an excellent source of selenium and copper, a very good source of zinc, and a good source of manganese, vitamin D (in the D2 form) and fibre.

I prefer to use shiitake Donko, traditionally grown in Japan, as it is one of the highest ranked, richest-tasting shiitake.

Dried Donko can be prepared for cooking by soaking them in water for about 2 hours. When soaked, Donko's flavour, aroma, vitamins and other substances (including eritadenin, an isolate of shiitake that helps lower blood pressure) are released into the soaking water. Therefore, it is recommended the soaking water be used to make stocks, soups, steamed dishes and sauces. It is believed that drinking soaking water every morning, heated as a tea, helps stabilise blood pressure and decrease cholesterol levels. It is not necessary to bring it to a boil before drinking.

Shiitake mushrooms can be used as an ingredient in miso soup (which I do), stir-fries, noodle dishes and stews.

Both fresh and dried best quality shiitake mushrooms are recommended.

SHOYU

Shoyu is the Japanese name for soy sauce, an all-purpose seasoning. I use traditional naturally fermented shoyu made from whole soybeans, wheat (used to grow the culture), natural sea salt and water. Commercially produced soy sauce takes only three to six months to ferment in artificially temperature-controlled vats, whereas my preferred shoyu is aged naturally for 18 to 24 months.

In 1254, a Buddhist priest named Kakushin from Wakayama Prefecture (western part of Japan) brought back the origin of soy sauce, miso 'Moromi', from China. Then he taught the people of the Wakayama area how to make soy sauce. The knowledge was then passed on to Shodo Island, which is located across the Inland Sea from Wakayama Prefecture, and from there spread across Japan.

Today, Shodo Island, unlike the other parts of Japan, remains pollution-free and is known for its natural picturesque views. The climate on this island, which at one time boasted over 400 individual soy sauce manufacturers, is ideally suited to soy sauce production. Soy sauce has now been produced on Shodo Island for over 400 years. In its pristine environment, one of Muso's soy sauces is manufactured, using only traditional methods handed down from one generation to the next. This is the shoyu made for Spiral Foods Australia and my favourite shoyu.

FYI: In the west, the terms shoyu and tamari are often used interchangeably. In Japan, shoyu is the soy sauce that is made from a mash of soybeans and wheat while tamari is a non-wheat product made by drawing off the liquid content of soybean miso.

SWEETENERS

All sweeteners should be used sparingly! All three sweeteners described below should be refrigerated or kept in a cool dry place after the seal is broken. They will last longer in the refrigerator.

Rice Syrup – Organic

This natural grain sweetener is derived by culturing cooked rice with enzymes to break down the starches, then straining off the liquid and reducing it by cooking until the desired consistency is reached. The final product contains soluble, slow-digesting carbohydrates, maltose and a small amount of glucose.

Rice syrup is mildly sweet – not as sweet as honey or sugar – with an almost butterscotch taste. It has a long history in Japan and was the traditional Japanese sweetener before the introduction of cane sugar. In ancient times, rice syrup was believed to be of divine origin. Rice was considered a gift of the gods, and its transformation into an ambrosial liquid sweetness was only allowed to take place in shrines and sacred places.

Traditional rice syrup is hard to find in modern Japan but is easy to find in Western natural food stores.

Maple Syrup – Organic

Maple syrup has been consumed for many centuries in North America, with 80 per cent of the world's supply now produced in Canada.

In cold climates, maple trees store starch in their trunks and roots before the winter. The starch is then converted to sugar that rises in the sap in late winter and early spring. Maple trees are tapped by drilling holes into their trunks and collecting the exuded sap, which is heat-processed to evaporate much of the water, leaving the concentrated syrup.

There are several different grades of maple syrup, which can be told apart by the colour. Grade B is the darkest with the strongest maple flavour.

The main thing that sets maple syrup apart from refined sugar is the fact that it also contains some minerals and antioxidants.

Coconut Syrup – Organic

This is a sweetener made from the nectar of coconut palm flowers. This nectar is found inside the blossoms of the coconut tree. Farmers tap the sweet nectar in a way similar to that of maple syrup production. It is then collected and placed under controlled evaporation until it reaches the consistency of syrup. With a distinctive sweet flavour, it can be used in all types of cooking.

'Overall, there isn't much difference between white table sugar and other natural sugars including coconut, honey, maple syrup (my personal favourite), molasses and sorghum. To the body, they are all sugar to be converted to glucose for metabolic fuel. But note that agave nectar can be 85 per cent fructose, while maple syrup is about 35 per cent.' Dr Andrew Weil, MD.

TAHINI (SESAME) PASTE

Tahini is a seed butter made from sesame seeds that are ground and toasted. It is commonly used in North African, Greek, Iranian, Turkish and Middle Eastern cuisine.

Tahini is high in protein and a rich source of B vitamins that boost energy and brain function; vitamin E, which is protective against heart disease and stroke; and important minerals, such as magnesium, iron and calcium.

Dark tahini, made from unhulled sesame, is strong tasting and slightly bitter, and perhaps slightly healthier, because many of the nutrients are in the husk. However, an alternative view is that the fibre in the husk impairs mineral absorption. I prefer the taste of the paler hulled tahini, made from hulled seeds and naturally organic. Either way, tahini is nutrient dense.

According to the USDA National Nutrient Database, a 2 tablespoon serving of tahini contains 178 calories, 16 grams of fat, 6 grams of carbohydrates (3 grams of fibre and 0 grams of sugar) and 5 grams of protein.

That same 2 tablespoon serving provides 30% of your daily thiamin needs, 24% of magnesium, 22% of phosphorus, 14% of iron and 12% of calcium.

Don't be alarmed by the amount of fat in tahini – only 2 out of the 16 grams are saturated while the rest are mono- and polyunsaturated fats, known to be beneficial to the heart and overall health.

TAMARI

Tamari was first produced as a by-product of soybean miso, when the people making the miso discovered the value of the raw liquid they drew off from the cedar kegs during the fermentation process. Since then, tamari itself has become a popular soy sauce product. The actual translation of tamari is 'puddle', so called for the way it would pool on top of the miso.

Since genuine tamari is a non-wheat product, it has a distinctive aroma as well as a thicker texture, deeper colour and stronger taste than shoyu (soy sauce).

TEMPEH

Tempeh is a fermented soybean food that originated in Indonesia, and is especially popular on the island of Java, where it is a staple source of protein. Like tofu, tempeh is made from soybeans, but it is a whole soybean product with different nutritional characteristics and textural qualities. A very different taste to tofu, tempeh has a textured and nutty flavour. Tempeh's fermentation process and its use of the whole bean give it a higher content of protein, fibre, vitamins (B vitamins and folate) and minerals such as iron and calcium. It is a probiotic food and low in saturated fats – but still containing essential fats. It has a firm texture and an earthy flavour that becomes more pronounced as it ages. It ferments with a natural fermentation starter for about 24 to 40 hours at around 30°C. This process binds the beans together, making a dense, white cake.

Once the fermentation process has finished, the tempeh is used as a raw ingredient in cooking.

When I lived in Bali, I really enjoyed eating vegetarian Nasi Campur (a mixed rice dish) and Gado Gado with tempeh. On my travels, I would often see soybeans being fermented in the sun.

TOFU

Tofu originated in China thousands of years ago. Legend has it that it was discovered about 2000 years ago by a Chinese cook who accidentally curdled soy milk when he added nigari seaweed.

Tofu, or bean curd, is made by curdling fresh soya milk, pressing it into a solid block and then cooling it – in much the same way that traditional dairy cheese is made by curdling and solidifying milk. The liquid (whey) is discarded when the curds are pressed into the gelatinous white blocks recognized as tofu.

Tofu is very low in cholesterol and sodium. It is also a good source of calcium, iron, magnesium, phosphorus and copper, and a very good source of protein, manganese and selenium. Tofu is naturally gluten free.

According to traditional Chinese medicine, tofu has a cooling character. It acts on the stomach, spleen and the large intestine and helps to clear the toxins (build-up of undigested food) in the intestine.

Soy bean products were traditionally used in China in very small quantities. Unfortunately, when people switch from dairy to soy products they consume soy in huge quantities. Soy bean products such as soy milk and tofu are considered cold damp in nature and can produce just as much phlegm and mucus in the throat as dairy. To reduce phlegm and mucus in the throat, eliminate soy-based products.

When buying tofu, to ensure the soybeans used to make tofu are not genetically modified, buy organic, which, by law, cannot contain genetically modified organisms.

When opened, all tofu needs to be rinsed, covered with water and kept in a refrigerated container. To keep the tofu fresh for up to one week, the water should be changed often.

Given its neutral taste and range of consistency, tofu has an amazing ability to work with almost all types of flavours and foods. Extra firm tofu is recommended for baking, grilling and stir-fries, while soft tofu is great for sauces, desserts, shakes and salad dressings.

Not recommended

Soy oil is highly refined, has an unpleasant intense aroma and flavour, is considered toxic in traditional Chinese medicine and it is difficult to digest. Unrefined soy oil is no better!

Soy cheese contains no cholesterol but does contain oil and may contain casein, a cow's milk derivative.

I don't encourage the use of hard-to-digest soy products that have not had the trypsin inhibitors removed. These include soy flour, soy grits, soy flakes, soy nuts and soy nut butter.

Also, super-refined soy products, such as lecithin, soy isolates, soy protein, TSP and TVP (both made from defatted soybeans using thermoplastic extrusion) are not recommended.

Purchase only certified organic foods or products with a manufacturer's statement that it uses no GMO, otherwise you are most probably ingesting Roundup Ready Soybeans spliced with a herbicide that enables the plant to survive other toxic doses of chemicals.

For those concerned about hypothyroidism and eating tofu, it is suggested that you eat cooked tofu in small amounts and make sure you are eating iodine-rich sea vegetables too. Read this article for more information:

Messina, M & Redmond, G 2006 'Effects of soy protein and soybean isoflavones on thyroid function in healthy adults and hypothyroid patients: a review of the relevant literature.' Thyroid, 16(3):249-58.

https://www.ncbi.nlm.nih.gov/pubmed/16571087

TURMERIC

Turmeric (Curcuma longa) is a member of the Zingiberaceae, or ginger, family, and, like ginger, is a tropical plant. Turmeric is native to tropical South Asia. You probably know turmeric as the main spice in curry. It has a warm, bitter taste and contains a yellow-coloured chemical called curcumin, which is frequently used to flavour or colour curry powders, mustards, butters, cheeses and even cosmetics. The root of turmeric is also used widely to make medicine.

In folk medicine, turmeric has traditionally been used to relieve liver problems, depression and stomach disorders and control diabetes. It was even thought to slow the ageing process.

Curcumin is a fat-soluble antioxidant. Research is underway that shows that curcumin and other chemicals in turmeric do seem to carry anti-inflammatory and anti-tumour properties. Because of this, turmeric might be beneficial for treating conditions that involve inflammation.

UMEBOSHI PLUMS

The umeboshi plum that I love to eat and use in all my classes is a traditional Japanese pickle. Unusually salty, sour and subtly sweet, they are great at helping you digest carbohydrates and proteins.

Ume means plum in Japanese, but they are actually a Japanese apricot.

The ume plant has been part of Japanese culture for centuries. Umeboshi plums were brought to Japan around 1500 years ago as a medicine, and their effectiveness was first documented in Chinese medicine books around 1500 years before that. The plums first became popular among priests and samurai warriors after the 12th century.

Fresh ume plums are very astringent and can't be eaten raw as they'll give you a tummy ache. But in salted pickled form, they're perfectly safe to eat and are quite delicious.

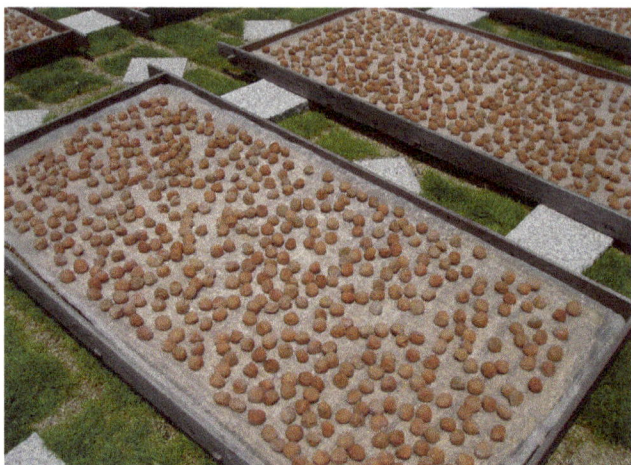
Drying umeboshi plums

According to Muso International Japan (the suppliers of my favourite Spiral Foods Organic Umeboshi), there is a traditional saying in Japan, 'Drink morning tea with umeboshi'. The reason behind this saying is that umeboshi contains citric acid, which helps sterilise the intestines while the stomach is empty in the morning. Also, the pyruvic acid in umeboshi helps activate the functions of various organs. Umeboshi has been an indispensable health tool for many years.

Also according to Muso International Japan, 'Organic acids in ume plums make the intestines temporarily acidic which prevents the live bacteria from increasing in number. After being absorbed through the wall of the intestines the organic acids become alkalized and enter the blood stream to maintain alkalized blood. With the help of this sterilizing effect, people have used Umeboshi as an ingredient inside rice balls and other foods for preservation'.

Highly alkaline ume from Japan are harvested by hand from June through July. After the harvest, they are pickled in salt for one month and sun-dried for three or four days. The sun-dried umeboshi are stored in kegs for about one year in order to balance the taste. Finally, they are pickled with shiso leaves and ume vinegar for colouring for a couple of weeks.

Traditionally, ume has been used in the following ways:

- For gastrointestinal ailments: stomach ache, diarrhoea, bad breath, constipation, indigestion, food poisoning, motion and morning sickness and other forms of nausea, and lack of appetite. (Sucking on the sour pit is an aid for neutralising acid reflux.)
- For antibiotic, antiseptic and anti-dysentery purposes.
- For fatigue, as they fight the harmful effects of excess lactic and pyruvic acid, which are the normal products of energy production in the body.
- As an antioxidant.
- For miscellaneous other purposes: anaemia, acne, headache, heatstroke, hangover, problems due to excess alcohol consumption, earache, colds and flu, and post-surgical recuperation.

Umeboshi vinegar is the juice extracted from making pickled umeboshi plums. It is the liquid that rises after the salt-soaked plums are pressed with stone weights. Although it is called plum vinegar, it is not true vinegar. Unlike brown rice vinegar, there is no acetic acid but instead plenty of citric acid, which lends it a relatively strong sourness.

How to use umeboshi

Umeboshi plums – Cook with grains, chew.

FYI: The shiso leaves used to give the red colour of ume are also known as perilla or beefsteak leaves.

Umeboshi puree – Mix into dips, drink in Kukicha twig tea.

Umeboshi vinegar – Use as a salad dressing or instead of brown rice vinegar for making sushi rice.

Ume Sho Bancha

A favourite macrobiotic home remedy to warm you up and alkalise and support your immune system.

- Brew kukicha twig tea according to instructions.
- Mash a half or whole umeboshi plum in a cup and mix well with 1 teaspoon (5 ml) of naturally brewed, organic Japanese shoyu or tamari.
- Pour boiling Kukicha twig tea into the cup and add a few drops of ginger juice. Serve hot.

VEGETABLES FROM THE SEA

Why would anyone want to eat sea vegetables? That was a big question when I started in the mid-1980s to use these traditional Japanese ingredients in my classes. Seaweed and marine algae have more concentrated nutrition than vegetables grown on land and they have long been considered to possess powers to prolong life, prevent disease, and impart beauty and health. For thousands of years, this mineral-rich vegetable has been a staple in Asian diets. Vegetables from the sea provide one of the broadest ranges of minerals of any food, containing nearly all the minerals found in the ocean and many of the same minerals found in human blood. There are measurable amounts of minerals such as calcium, copper, iodine, iron, magnesium, manganese, molybdenum, phosphorus, potassium, selenium, vanadium and zinc. They are also high in antioxidants and packed with vitamins A, C, E, B complex and B12. In addition, edible seaweeds provide protein, fibre and even some omega-3 fatty acids.

I store my sea vegetables in an airtight container in a cool place and, when opened, in my fridge. I use traditional Japanese arame in salads and stir-fries, wakame in soups and salads, yakinori for nori rolls and snacks, Furikake sea vegetable shake and dulse flakes as garnish, agar for desserts and, even though it is hard to buy in Australia, kombu. Read more about each seaweed in their individual glossary entries.

WAKAME SEA VEGETABLE

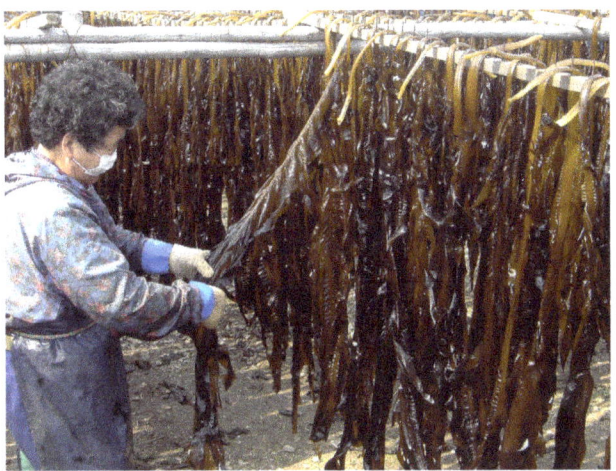
Drying wakame   Photo: Muso International Japan

Wakame is a dark green leaf used in soups, salads, stews and casseroles. It is an annual sea vegetable that grows on rocks as deep as three to ten metres under the sea. I prefer wakame that is hand harvested and dried under the sun.

Wakame has the smell of the sea and a dark green colour. Besides miso soup, wakame also is suited for steamed vegetables and salads. Wakame will be dark green and softer if you boil it lightly after soaking in water. It is important to soak and boil it only for short time, otherwise the texture, colour and flavour will be poor. When using in miso soup, it is best to add at the end of cooking time. When using in vinegared dishes, add wakame last as the colour and flavour will be so much better.

WASABI

I use and recommend Spiral Foods Natural Wasabi Powder which is a pale, green horseradish-like paste made from a semi-aquatic wild plant of the cabbage family. It is made from horseradish, spirulina and turmeric. Mix a small amount of hot water with a little powder to make a thick paste. Allow the paste to rest for a minute to release its fiery qualities.

FYI: You should know that the commercially packaged green wasabi paste that is served with sushi isn't really wasabi. It is a combination of sorbitol, glucose, corn starch, horseradish, mustard, wheat, food colouring, and preservatives.

Real wasabi root, if you can find it, is both pungent and much more flavourful than the fake stuff. In addition, genuine wasabi has interesting therapeutic effects, including antibiotic properties (which may be one reason Japanese have traditionally used it as a condiment for raw fish). Wasabi aids digestion, works as a germicide and helps clear the sinuses.

It is an excellent addition to marinades, dips and dressings.

VOODLES

These are vegetables spiralled or peeled to resemble noodles. With a vegetable of your choice (carrots, cucumber, zucchini etc.), simply glide your peeler vertically downwards to create thin shavings or 'voodles'. This can also be done using a spiraliser tool if you have one (I love my Japanese-made vegetable turner/shredder). Strips made out of zucchini have their own term, 'zoodles'.

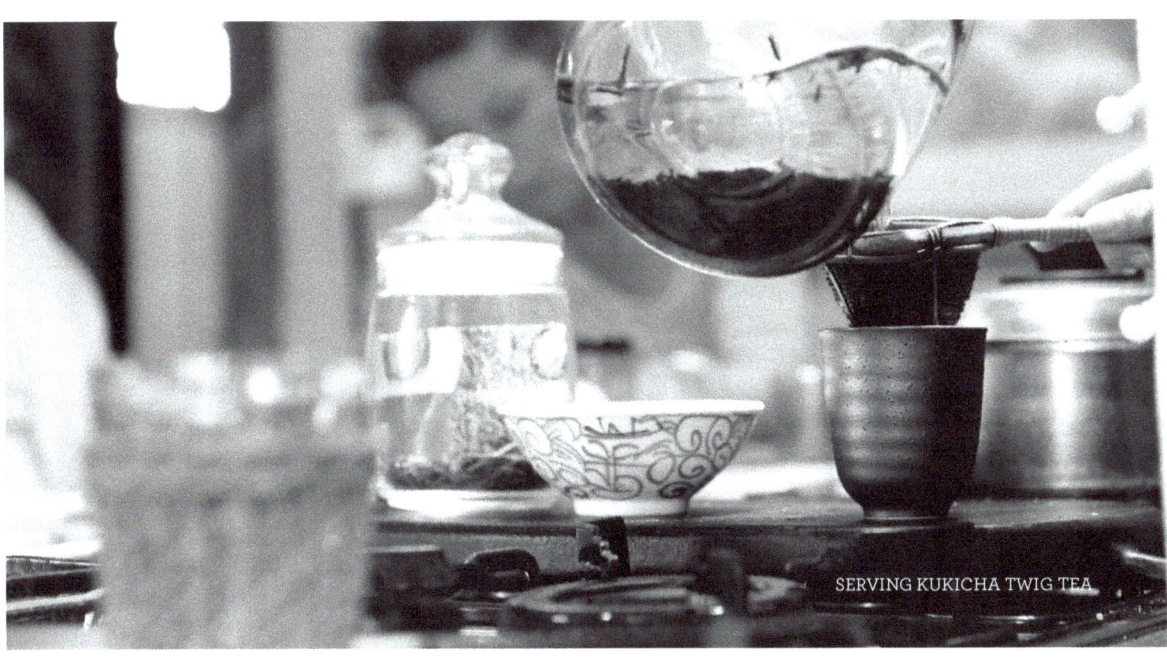
SERVING KUKICHA TWIG TEA

MY WHOLEFOOD JOURNEY

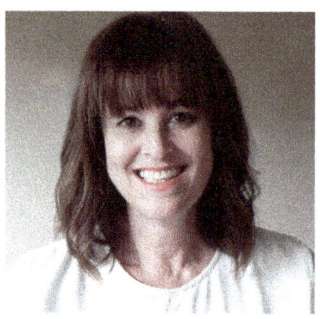

This book has been a long time in the making: just ask the many people who have come to my wholefood cooking and nutrition classes over the past 30 years. Almost daily, someone asks me for a copy of my cookbook and I have to reply, 'It's a work in progress'. As with most creative ventures, a book needs time to gestate. Finally, the time has come to share my experience and knowledge in print.

In the past couple of years, I have been gathering feedback from past students as to their favourite recipes, crowdfunding the money to self-publish, selecting recipes, cooking and testing again and again, and getting all the recipes professionally photographed from cooking to plate. It was very important to me that the photos were taken in my own kitchen with no food photography tricks as I want you to see how the finished recipes will look when you make them.

I am so thankful and blessed to have good friends in my community who are professional photographers, designers, chefs, IT geeks and food lovers. I appreciate so much the support from my family, friends and community that has enabled me to publish this book.

My Wholefood Community Cook Book is the culmination of my years of passion and interest in using plant-based wholefoods as medicines that were initially motivated by the desire to improve and maintain my own health after an early medical challenge. I committed myself to supporting myself and others in the quest to live a healthy lifestyle and prevent illness and dis-ease. Prevention is a key element of my philosophy. An especially meaningful component of my work is supporting people with digestive disorders, food intolerances, inflammation and cancer through specific classes and consultations, which I was able to develop based on my own experiences and studies.

I am a very private person and I never wanted to lead my career with the 'I am a survivor' banner, but I am now ready to share my personal story in the hope that it may inspire, educate and comfort others.

In 1977, at the age of 20, I developed Hodgkin's lymphoma, a cancer of the lymphatic system, which forms part of the immune system. To treat it, I had to have my spleen removed. The spleen is an important part of the immune system and contains special white blood cells that destroy bacteria and help your body fight infections when you are sick. It also acts as a purifier for the blood, removing microbes and worn-out or damaged red blood cells from the body's circulation. After this splenectomy, I underwent intensive radiotherapy and suffered from side effects including nausea, vomiting, hair loss and fatigue.

Fortunately, the treatment worked and the cancer was eradicated but my immune system was forever compromised. In addition, remission is only declared after five years so my health challenge remained at the front of my mind and spurred on my interest in foods as medicines and eliminating foods that would compromise my immune system.

Thankfully, many people, including myself, enjoy long and healthy lives after being successfully treated for Hodgkin's lymphoma. Sometimes, however, the treatment can affect a person's health for months or even years after it has finished. These effects are called long-term or late effects and may include fertility problems and a higher risk of developing a secondary cancer later in life.

I didn't discover the benefits of health foods immediately after my initial diagnosis and I can't honestly say that I cured myself with plant-based wholefoods at the time. However, I knew that I could help my immune system and improve the quality of my life by changing and improving my diet from then on.

I decided, from investigations, to be a vegetarian but I didn't really know how to get balanced nutrition from vegetarian foods. It was the mid-1980s and, without the internet, information about the medicinal benefits of food was hard to find. Back then, there were no 'superfoods' and organic foods were not readily available but it was possible to eat a simple plant-based diet and I soon discovered that I really began to feel better eating this way. I did feel that I was remedying my ailments with foods and herbs. That was my awakening into using foods as medicines. My immune system improved, my mood improved and even my hair grew back shiny and thick and I began to feel rejuvenated. I learnt to pace myself better, I felt calmer and I began to sleep well.

I needed to find out more about how to maintain a healthy diet. I began to spend more time with people who were vegetarians and interested in herbs and natural remedies and I loved going into health food stores. I also started reading a lot about vegetarianism and macrobiotics and attending short courses at the local naturopathic school.

It was at this stage that I found my interest in cooking beginning to grow. The kitchen had always been the real heart of our family home but I had never considered cooking as a career. Instead, by then, I had degrees in Business Accounting and Marketing and was working as an accountant and on the side cooking for friends and a few clients.

I embraced my new-found passion and trusted my instincts! I eventually left my well-paid accounting job to work in a health food store in Melbourne. The owner, Margaret Barrett, an extraordinary woman, taught me so much and was a huge influence.

In the 1980s, Australia was way behind the rest of the world when it came to macrobiotics and natural and organic foods. I discovered so much when I travelled to the USA and Europe during that decade. I went to every possible workshop and seminar to learn from those who came before me in the health food movement, including Annemarie Colbin at the Natural Gourmet Institute in New York, and Herman and Cornelia Aihara and David and Cynthia Briscoe in California. It is thanks to these pioneers that we know so much about alkalising, plant-based nutrient-rich medicinal wholefoods.

Meeting Michio Kushi, one of the founders of macrobiotics, when he came to Melbourne at the end of the 1980s also had a huge impact on me. Because of him, I learnt to focus on eating a wider variety of plant-based foods. He would specially joke with me and point out when I did not chew my food properly so I also learnt about the benefits of chewing (so important for digestive health).

By 1985, I was managing a well-known large health food store and cafe, Soulfood South Yarra. This store was one of the loves of my life. It was way ahead of its time for sure and I spent a lot of my time educating as well as feeding my customers. One of my regulars was James Wilson of Spiral Foods, who, in 1986, invited me to work at Spiral Foods as a sales representative and to assist with marketing. While there, I embraced the opportunity to learn as much as possible about traditional Japanese medicinal foods and Spiral Foods' natural and macrobiotic products.

By then I had been to many cooking classes but in 1987 the student became the teacher when James and I started a traditional Japanese cooking school, the first of its kind in Melbourne. Our aim was to educate people in traditional Japanese and macrobiotic ingredients at a time when there were only about six Japanese restaurants around. We joined forces with Osamu Ito (Itosan), a master Japanese chef, and invited many top macrobiotic and vegetarian cooking teachers, to teach at our school.

I bought Soulfood and changed the name to Manna Natural Foods Store in 1988. I stocked a wide variety of grocery items, organic dried herbs and supplements. I also had a small café that was popular with those who were already aware of healthy eating – lots of overseas actors and musicians – and for a few years my store was the unofficial health food store for tennis players who came to play the Australian Open. (No name dropping here.)

I loved that store and especially its many wonderful customers but running the health food store and the café on my own was too challenging for me and my constitution. The store needed renovation, new equipment and more help and, on advice and with a heavy heart, I had to close. I was devastated for several months.

Thankfully, a few months later, I was given the opportunity to set up and run the Health Café and Juice Bar at Daimaru Department Store. It was the first of its kind in the Melbourne CBD and was a great success until changes were made at Daimaru that led to it closing.

At this stage, the early 1990s, I left Melbourne to live in Bali and was able to continue to teach vegetarian and macrobiotic cooking. It was very inspiring to live there as I discovered a shared interest in creativity, food, spirituality, local traditions and, for sure, having a great time. However, the tropical Balinese climate had an effect on my immune system, so after nearly two years, I had to return to live in Melbourne.

After my return I discovered I had a growth on my thyroid and unfortunately had to have half of it removed. I had always suspected that radiation treatment raises the risk of other forms of cancer in the part of the body that received radiation. This suspicion – which has since been medically proven – was confirmed for me by the discovery of this thyroid growth.

In 2002, I had the great opportunity to study with medical practitioners and natural therapists in Swinburne University's Graduate Diploma of Applied Science in Nutritional and Environmental Medicine. Professor Avni Sali AM created the course to educate practitioners in evidence-based complementary and alternative medicines and to emphasise the principles and practical application of nutritional and environmental medicine to common clinical problems. These studies – and my associations with pioneers in the art and science of wellbeing and healing – were a most thrilling and inspiring experience for me and encouraged me even more to continue educating, counselling and sharing with people in my cooking classes and seminars. Given my own health challenges, I truly understand that knowledge is power, and I love that I am able to empower others.

Due to my medical history, I was always diligent about having check-ups every two years. In 2012, it was discovered that I had a really small tumour in my breast. After consulting many cancer specialists, both conventional and alternative, I decided to have a double mastectomy and reconstruction to prevent further breast tumours from occurring due to the radiation damage from all those years ago. It was the best decision for me. It was a huge operation, rendering me horizontal for weeks and in recovery for several more weeks, plus three further reconstructive operations over the next couple of years.

It was certainly a difficult time. I only shared my situation with my family and a few close friends as I didn't want to attract a lot of attention or sympathy. I knew that I had to do what I felt was needed and to focus on my own treatment, which my knowledge and experience had given me the power and necessary tools to do. It was best for me not to tune into the advice and stories from many well-meaning people and especially their often-fearful views of cancer. I felt that having to explain my situation would be draining for me and my nearest and dearest. I was also keen to continue working and I didn't want my personal situation to detract from supporting my clients and students or even my social life.

After successful recovery many years ago, I am doing and being really well. I am able to maintain my healthy attitude by nourishing myself with plant-based wholefoods, exercise, good times and eliminating stress and negative energy.

Cooking has always been a kind of meditative practice for me so this continues to be a great help. Food is my medicine on so many levels.

Using food to aid healing involves a conscious decision and total commitment but my healthy lifestyle really supported my recovery each and every time I encountered a new health challenge, and for that, and all those who've taught me along the way, I'm grateful.

For over thirty years, my friends, clients and I have eaten and continue to eat the delicious recipes that I'm now sharing with you in *My Wholefood Community Cookbook*. These recipes reflect the greatest prescription for good health. Take care of you. Eat well. Be well.

Good health, naturally,
Sandra

Melbourne, Australia 2018.
Wholefood Nutrition, Natural Food Consultant
& Cooking Teacher.

Bachelor of Business (Accounting) RMIT
Bachelor of Business (Marketing) Monash University
Graduate Diploma of Applied Science in Nutritional and Environmental Medicine, Swinburne University
Certificate IV in Training and Assessment, Box Hill Institute
Certificate III in Hospitality (Commercial Cookery), Holmesglen Institute
Macrobiotic Health Training USA

   www.mywholefoodcommunity.com
   @mywholefoodcommunity

MY FAVOURITE RESOURCES

COOKWARE & KITCHEN UTENSILS

- Airtight glass jars
- Bamboo steamers
- Bamboo sushi mats
- Benriner Japanese Horizontal Turning Slicer
- Cast iron woks – small and large
- Japanese pickle Press
- Japanese porcelain ginger grater
- Japanese suribachi and surikogi (Japanese mortar and pestle)
- Le Creuset stoneware and cast iron cookware
- Magimix food processor
- My mother's 50 year old cast iron frypan
- Stainless steel knives – my favourite is my well used Japanese Caddie knife
- Stick blender
- Vintage Pyrex heat-resistant glass teapot (used in all my cooking classes to boil and serve Kukicha twig tea)
- Vitamix and Ladyship high-speed blenders
- Waters Co purifying Bio Ace Alkaline Mineral Pot and Waterman Portable Alkaline Water filter (which I especially like to take on my travels)
- Wooden and bamboo chopping boards and cooking utensils

PUBLICATIONS

- Books and training at Natural Gourmet Institute NYC and Annemarie Colbin
- Books and training by Michio and Aveline Kushi
- Books and training by Herman and Cornelia Aihara
- Books by Dean Ornish
- Books and website by Dr Andrew Weil
- Books and television programmes by Michael Mosley
- Macrobiotics America – David & Cynthia Briscoe
- Mayo Clinic website
- Nutrition Australia website
- The World's Healthiest Foods website
- *Eat, Drink, and Be Healthy: The Harvard Medical School Guide To Healthy Eating* – Walter C. Willett, M.D.
- *Let Food Be Thy Medicine* – Alex Jack
- *The Blue Zones: Lessons for Living Longer from the People Who've Lived the Longest* – Dan Buettner
- *Healing With Whole Foods* – Paul Pitchford
- *Herbs and Natural Supplements: An Evidence-Based Guide* – Prof. Leslie Braun & Prof. Marc Cohen
- *The Truth About Food* – Jill Fullerton-Smith
- *Nature's Cancer-Fighting Foods* – Verne Varona
- *The New Whole Foods Encyclopedia* – Rebecca Wood
- *Whole: Rethinking Science of Nutrition* – T. Colin Campbell PhD
- *In Defence Of Food & The Omnivore's Dilemma* – Michael Pollan

DOCUMENTARIES

- Food Matters
- Food Inc
- A Delicate Balance
- Forks Over Knives
- Hungry For Change
- That Sugar Film
- Michael Pollan – Cooked & Food Fight

ACKNOWLEDGEMENTS

Inspirational community, teachers and mentors

- Annemarie Colbin – Natural Gourmet Institute, New York, USA
- Michio Kushi – Kushi Institute, USA
- Herman and Cornellia Aihara – Macrobiotics America
- David and Cynthia Briscoe – Macrobiotics America
- James Wilson – Spiral Foods Australia
- Margaret and Don Barrett – they owned the first health food store I worked at in 1985.
- Professor Avni Sali – National Institute of Integrative Medicine, Australia
- Professor Ian Brighthope – Nutrition Care Pharmaceuticals, Australia
- Professor Marc Cohen – RMIT University Health Innovations Research Institute, Australia. We have had many wonderful experiences teaching medical students about food as medicine and travelling to holistic health conferences overseas
- Master Chef Osamu Ito (who I fondly and respectfully call Itosan) has been a great teacher of traditional Japanese cuisine to me and many others. We have had many wonderful experiences together in cooking classes and large public food festivals over the last 30 years
- Master Chef Jitendra Bhatia, who founded Vegetable Creations in 1987 (handmade delicious and healthy, certified organic vegetarian products) has shared not only a vegetarian café with me but also Ayurvedic knowledge and organic vegetarian cooking principles. It's very special that we have, aside from sharing good food over many years, shared good times and good friendship
- Brinthapan Parathan – Information Technology advisor and webmaster, great photographer and supporter of this project
- All the extraordinary conventional and integrative medical practitioners, natural therapists, spiritual teachers, health food retailers and wholesalers, students and clients I have had the privilege of meeting, working together and supporting.

My Wholefood Community Cookbook team

- Gabrielle Hagan – assistant in all my cooking classes for the past 10 years and a true friend who has greatly encouraged me to get this book done and especially helped to chop, wash dishes and cook all the food for this book. Gabe is my angel who especially was there for me and rose to the task of caring for me and cooking my plant based wholefood recipes in my own times of need.
- Emmanuel Santos – a Melbourne-based documentary and art photographer, whose work is found in dozens of museum collections both here and overseas. Photos were taken in natural lighting as each recipe was cooked and plated.
- Russel Bradley – The Hive Design, the great studio responsible for design and layout of this book.
- Irene Metter – The Hive Design, who, since designing my first cooking video material in 1999 and all my marketing designs ever since, is a great friend, my passionate supporter, lover of my food and, though she has many projects as a documentary film maker, has found the time to typeset this book.
- Stephanie Heriot AE – my delightful editor who thankfully has really good ideas and an eye for detail.

Special thanks go to Mercantile Home Melbourne for providing the high quality, uniquely designed tableware photographed in *My Wholefood Community Cookbook*.

Thanks so much to Waters Co Australia for ensuring that I always have access to clean, great tasting, and alkaline mineral water. These water filters remove bacteria, harmful chemicals and heavy metals while adding minerals such as magnesium and calcium to the water. During all my cooking classes and seminars we drink and cook with super hydrating, anti-oxidant, purified, alkaline mineral water from Waters Co Australia.

Much appreciation to Muso International Japan, the traditional Japanese organic foods and macrobiotics food trader, for photos of product making processes.

Crowdfunding support – I couldn't have made *My Wholefood Community Cookbook* happen without the great advice from staff at Pozible in Collingwood, Melbourne. Crowdfunding is a wonderful opportunity to self-publish. I went to all seminars that they ran over a year and asked many questions before I felt ready to give crowdfunding a go and thankfully it worked out.

My Pantry Essentials

SOYFOODS	SEA VEGETABLES	ORGANIC OILS
Miso	Arame	Sesame – toasted
Shoyu	Wakame, Kombu	Sesame – natural
Tamari	Sushi Nori	Extra virgin olive
Tofu	Agar Agar	Coconut
Tempeh	Dulse flakes	
	Sesame and Sea Vegetable seasoning	

ORGANIC WHOLEGRAINS	ORGANIC BEANS	ORGANIC TEAS
Brown rice	Adzuki, Black, Pinto, Kidney	Kukicha twig
Hulled millet	Chickpea	Green
Quinoa	Green & Red lentils, Split peas	Herbals
Oats	Urad Dal, Chana Dal	Dandelion
Buckwheat	Organic beans BPA free tin	

SEASONINGS	EXTRAS	SWEETENERS
Umeboshi plums	Kuzu	Rice syrup
Umeboshi vinegar	Tahini	Coconut syrup
Brown rice vinegar	Shiitake mushroom	Maple syrup
Mirin	Pickles	Organic vanilla extract/pods
Apple cider vinegar	Udon, Soba, Sweet Potato, Rice noodles	Raw cacao
	Chickpea flour (Besan)	Coconut milk
	Tofu pouches (Abura Age)	Coconut, grated
	Smoked tofu	
	Tortilla flour (Masa Harina)	

HERBS AND SPICES	VEGETABLES	FRUITS
Basil, bay leaf, black pepper, caraway, cinnamon, cloves, coriander, cumin, curry, dill, garlic, ginger, oregano, parsley, thyme, vanilla	A colourful variety of organic greens and vegetables	In season – colourful variety Organic dried fruits

NUTS AND SEEDS	YOUR PANTRY ESSENTIALS	
Walnuts		
Almonds		
Cashews		
Hazelnuts		
Brazil nuts		
Sunflower		
Sesame		
Pumpkin		

INDEX

A
Adzuki bean spread 41
Adzuki bean vegetable stew 101
Almond satay sauce 43
Aquafaba meringues 144
Avocado
Broccoli avocado soup 22
Brown rice sushi rolls – norimaki 59
Noodle nori rolls 113
Raw beetroot avocado spread 41

B
Baked beetroot, grilled snake bean & fennel 69
Baked vegetable noodles (voodles) 73
Beans
Adzuki bean spread 41
Adzuki bean vegetable stew 101
Black bean Aztec salad 109
Kidney bean salad 97
Latin American quinoa bean soup 31
Quinoa black bean patties 89
Slow cooked spicy black bean & rice soup 33
Tex-Mex pinto bean dip 40
Beetroot
Baked beetroot, grilled snake bean & fennel 69
Red lentil beetroot soup 27
Tofu beetroot dip 39
Bircher muesli 149
Black bean Aztec salad 109
Broccoli avocado soup 22
Broccoli pancakes 77
Broccoli
Broccoli avocado soup 22
Broccoli pancakes 77
Vegetable noodle (voodle) stir fry 71
Brown rice for sushi 83
Brown rice porridge 150
Brown rice sushi rolls – norimaki 59
Brown rice vegetable paella 87
Buckwheat chickpea tabbouleh 93
Buckwheat
Buckwheat chickpea tabbouleh 93

C
Cabbage
Naturally pressed pickle salad 47
Pickled cabbage 49
Rice or bean noodle salad 119
Soba noodle stir fry 115
Carrot
Adzuki bean vegetable stew 101
Baked vegetable noodles (voodles) 73
Moroccan chickpea carrot tagine 98
Naturally pressed pickle salad 47
Noodle nori rolls 113
Slow cooked spicy black bean & rice soup 33
Sweet and sour arame 51
Sweet and sour quick pickles 49
Thai tofu vegetable patties 103
Tofu pouches – inari sushi 85
Tofu scramble – san choy bau 105
Vegetable noodle (voodle) stir fry 71
Wakame miso soup 21
Cashew 'cheese' sauce 73
Cauliflower
Millet cauliflower mash 80
Chiang mai vegetable noodle 121
Chickpea celery hummus 40
Chickpea polenta 102
Chickpea
Aquafaba meringues 144
Broccoli pancakes 77
Brown rice vegetable paella 87
Buckwheat chickpea tabbouleh 93
Chickpea celery hummus 40
Chickpea polenta 103
Kale almond pancakes 77
Moroccan chickpea carrot tagine 98
Zucchini pancakes 75
Chocolate almond fudge 135

Chocolate bark 139
Cocoa
Chocolate almond fudge 135
Chocolate bark 139
Ginger chocolate chip cookies 134
Homemade chocolate 145
Panforte slice 141
Raw cacao protein energy balls 145
Raw chocolate mousse 135
Sweet potato brownies 133
Coconut buttercream icing 133
Coconut chia almond pudding 148
Coconut chutney 127
Coconut tofu snake beans 63
Compote of dried fruits with nut cream 149
Cooking brown rice 82
Cooking hulled millet 80
Corn tortillas and taco shells 128
Corn
Black bean Aztec salad 109
Corn tortillas and taco shells 128
Latin American quinoa bean soup 31
Quinoa corn arame salad 91
Thai tofu vegetable patties 103
Creamy ginger dressing 57
Creamy quinoa pudding 151
Cucumber wakame salad 57
Cucumber wakame salad marinade 57

D
Dal vada – lentil fritters 107

G
Ginger apple pear sauce 134
Ginger chocolate chip cookies 134
Granola bars 136
Green miso pesto 38

H
Homemade chocolate 145
Homemade nut mylk 132

K

Kale almond pancakes 77
Kale chips 66
Kale miso soup 19
Kale
 Baked beetroot, grilled snake bean & fennel 69
 Kale almond pancakes 77
 Kale chips 66
 Kale miso soup 19
 Naturally pressed pickle salad 47
 Simply boiled kale with creamy ginger dressing 57
 Sweet potato noodle stir fry 117
Kidney bean salad 97
Kukicha twig tea 124

L

Latin American quinoa bean soup 31
Lentil walnut paté 36
Lentil
 Coconut chutney 127
 Dal vada – lentil fritters 107
 Lentil walnut paté 36
 Masala dosa 127
 Plain dosa 125
 Red lentil beetroot soup 27
 Slow cooked curried dahl 107
Lime vinaigrette 42

M

Masala dosa 127
Millet cauliflower mash 80
Millet
 Cooking hulled millet 80
 Millet cauliflower mash 80
 North African millet soup 29
 Pumpkin millet seed balls 81
 Soft millet porridge 150
Miso dill dressing 42
Miso tahini lemon sauce 36
Miso teriyaki paste 43
Miso umeboshi sauce 38
Miso
 Adzuki bean spread 41
 Cucumber wakame salad 57
 Green miso pesto 38
 Kale miso soup 19
 Kidney bean salad 97
 Lentil walnut paté 36
 Miso dill dressing 42
 Miso tahini lemon sauce 36
 Miso teriyaki paste 43
 Miso umeboshi sauce 38
 Quinoa corn arame salad 91
 Simply boiled kale with creamy ginger dressing 57
 Vegetable noodle (voodle) stir fry 71
 Wakame miso soup 21
 Moroccan chickpea carrot tagine 98
Mushroom
 Chiang mai vegetable noodles 121
 Kale miso soup 19
 Quinoa corn arame salad 91
 Shiitake sesame vinaigrette 42
 Soba noodle stir fry 115
 Sweet and sour arame 51
 Sweet potato noodle stir fry 117
 Thai tofu vegetable patties 103
 Tofu pouches – inari sushi 85
 Tofu scramble – san choy bau 105
 Wakame miso soup 21

N

Naturally pressed pickle salad 47
Noodle nori rolls 113
Nori pyramids – onigiri 61
North African millet soup 29
Nut-free crunchy quinoa brittle 141
Nuts
 Almond satay sauce 43
 Baked vegetable noodles (voodles) 73
 Chocolate almond fudge 135
 Chocolate bark 139
 Coconut chia almond pudding 148
 Compote of dried fruits with nut cream 149
 Ginger chocolate chip cookies 134
 Granola bars 136
 Green miso pesto 38
 Homemade chocolate 145
 Homemade nut mylk 132
 Kale almond pancakes 77
 Lentil walnut paté 36
 Panforte slice 141
 Sweet potato brownies 133
 Ted's oat granola 148
 Thai tofu vegetable patties 103

P

Panforte slice 141
Pear tart 142
Pickled cabbage 49
Pickles
 Naturally pressed pickle salad 47
 Pickled cabbage 49
 Sweet and sour arame 51
 Sweet and sour quick pickles 49
Plain dosa 125
Plum basil dressing 52
Pumpkin millet seed balls 81
Pumpkin
 Adzuki bean vegetable stew 101
 North African millet soup 29
 Pumpkin millet seed balls 81
 Split pea soup with smoked tofu 25

Q

Quinoa black bean patties 89
Quinoa corn arame salad 91
Quinoa
 Creamy quinoa pudding 151
 Latin American quinoa bean soup 31

Nut-free crunch quinoa brittle 141
Quinoa black bean patties 89
Quinoa corn arame salad 91

R

Raw beetroot avocado spread 41
Raw cacao protein energy balls 145
Raw chocolate mousse 135
Red curry paste 43
Red lentil beetroot soup 27
Rice or bean noodle salad 119

Rice
Brown rice for sushi 83
Brown rice porridge 150
Brown rice sushi rolls – norimaki 59
Brown rice vegetable paella 87
Cooking brown rice 82
Nori pyramids – onigiri 61
Sea vegetable brown rice 82
Slow cooked spicy black bean & rice soup 33
Tofu pouches – inari sushi 85

S

Sandy's seed mix 124
Sea vegetable brown rice 82

Sea vegetable
Brown rice for sushi 83
Cucumber wakame salad 57
Kidney bean salad 97
Nori pyramids – onigiri 61
Quinoa corn arame salad 91
Sea vegetable brown rice 82
Spring salad 52
Sweet and sour arame 51
Thai tofu vegetable patties 103
Wakame miso soup 21

Sesame dressing 55
Shiitake sesame vinaigrette 42
Simply boiled kale with creamy ginger dressing 57
Slow cooked curried dahl 107
Slow cooked spicy black bean & rice soup 33

Soba noodle stir fry 115
Soft millet porridge 150
Spinach roll with sesame dressing 55
Split pea soup with smoked tofu 25

Split pea
Slow cooked curried dahl 107
Split pea soup wih smoked tofu 25
Spring salad 52

Sweet and sour arame 51
Sweet and sour quick pickles 49
Sweet potato brownies 133
Sweet potato noodle stir fry 117

Sweet potato
Kale miso soup 19
North African millet soup 29
Slow cooked curried dahl 107
Sweet potato brownies 133
Sweet potato noodle stir fry 117
Thai tofu sweet potato curry 105
Thai tofu vegetable patties 103

Sweet tahini apple cider dressing 69

T

Ted's oat granola 148
Tempeh and tofu mustard 109
Tex-Mex pinto bean dip 40
Thai tofu sweet potato curry 105
Thai tofu vegetable patties 103
Thai vegetable stock 17
Tofu beetroot dip 39
Tofu pouches – inari sushi 85
Tofu scramble – san choy bau 105
Tofu sour cream 75

Tofu
Coconut tofu snake beans 63
Split pea soup wih smoked tofu 25
Tempeh and tofu mustard 109
Thai tofu sweet potato curry 105
Thai tofu vegetable patties 103
Tofu beetroot dip 39
Tofu pouches – inari sushi 85
Tofu scramble – san choy bau 105
Zucchini pancakes 75

U

Ume tahini dressing 47

Umeboshi
Adzuki bean spread 41
Lentil walnut paté 36
Miso umeboshi sauce 38
Nori pyramids – onigiri 61
Plum basil dressing 52

V

Vegetable noodle (voodle) stir fry 71
Vegetable stock 16

W

Wakame miso soup 21
White miso sauce 71

Z

Zucchini pancakes 75

Zucchini
Baked vegetable noodles (voodles) 73
Vegetable noodle (voodle) stir fry 71
Zucchini pancakes 75

MWC WEIGHTS AND MEASURES CONVERSIONS

When using a recipe from another country, know that standard measuring utensils vary. Australia uses metrics as the standard for measuring and some of the measuring utensils differ too. For example, the standard cup used in Australian cooking is 250 ml, 1 cup in Japan is 200 ml and in American 1 cup is 240 ml.
1 Australian tablespoon is 20 ml however North America, New Zealand and United Kingdom use 15 ml tablespoons.

This book uses Australian weights and measures.

WEIGHTS

GRAMS	OUNCES (approximate)
15 g	½ oz
30 g	1 oz
125 g	4 oz (¼ lb)
250 g (¼ kg)	8 oz (½ lb)
500 g (½ kg)	16 oz (1 lb)
1000 g (1 kg)	32 oz (2 lb)

VOLUME

METRIC	STANDARD MEASURES	IMPERIAL
20 ml	1 tbsp	½ fl oz
30 ml	1½ tbsp	1 fl oz
100 ml	5 tbsp	3 fl oz
250 ml	1 cup	8 fl oz
1.25 litres	5 cups	40 fl oz (1 quart)

LENGTH

METRIC	IMPERIAL (approximate)
5 mm	.2 inch
10 mm (1 cm)	.4 inch
20 mm (2 cm)	.8 inch
2.5 cm	1 inch
5 cm	2 inches
10 cm	4 inches

CUP MEASURES

	METRIC	IMPERIAL
1 cup flour	140 g	4½ oz
1 cup honey	375 g	12 oz
1 cup rice, uncooked	220 g	7 oz
1 cup nuts, chopped	125 g	4 oz

LIQUIDS

Cup measures

¼ cup = 60 ml

1 cup = 250 ml

4 cups = 1 litre = 1000 ml

4 cups = 1 quart

SPOON MEASURES

1 tablespoon = 20 ml

1 teaspoon = 5 ml

4 teaspoons = 1 tablespoon

SPOON WEIGHT MEASURES

1 level teaspoon = 5 g

1 level tablespoon = 20 g

OVEN TEMPERATURE

Oven temperatures are expressed in degrees Celsius (°C) or in Fahrenheit (°F) for gas and electric ovens. All oven types vary and the manufactures hand book should therefore be followed for correct usage. All ovens should be pre-heated before use to allow correct cooking times expressed and ensure product is cooked correctly.

All recipes in this book were tested using a fan-forced oven. If you are using a conventional oven, the rough rule of thumb is to add 10–20°C to the recommended temperature. Every oven behaves differently, so factor in your knowledge of your own oven. The temperatures provided are a guide only.

	GAS		ELECTRIC	
	CELSIUS	FAHRENHEIT	CELSIUS	FAHRENHEIT
Slow	120–135°C	250–275°F	120–150°C	250–300°F
Moderately slow	150–160°C	300–320°F	150–160°C	300–325°F
Moderate	175°C	350°F	175–205°C	350–400°F
Moderately hot	190°C	375°F	220–230°C	425–450°F
Hot	205–230°C	400–450°F	245–260°C	475–500°F
Very hot	245–260°C	475–500°F	275–290°C	525–550°F

Good health, naturally

www.ingramcontent.com/pod-product-compliance
Lightning Source LLC
Chambersburg PA
CBHW040729020526
44107CB00086B/2991